THE ART OF TANTRIC SEX

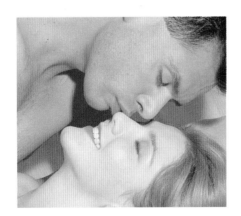

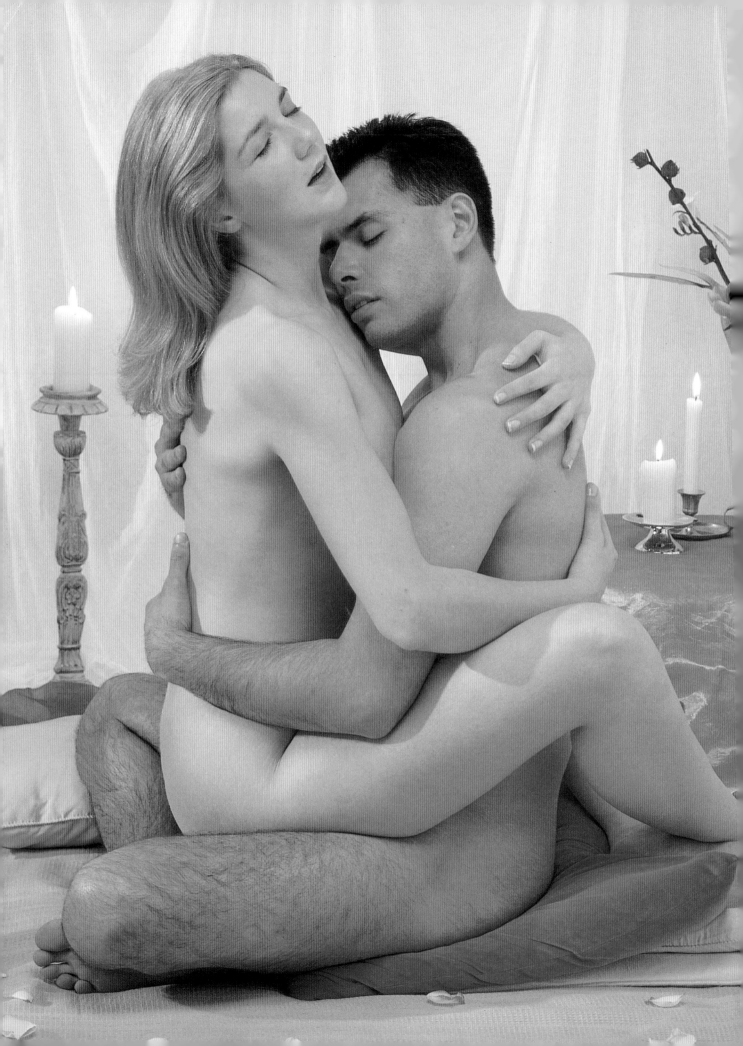

THE ART OF TANTRIC SEX

NITYA LACROIX

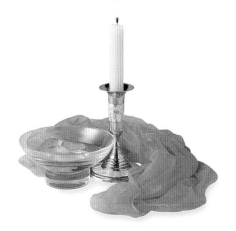

Photography by MARK HARWOOD

DK PUBLISHING, INC.

LONDON, NEW YORK, MUNICH,
MELBOURNE, AND DELHI

PROJECT EDITOR Damien Moore
PROJECT ART EDITOR Sharon Moore
US EDITOR Mary Sutherland
DESIGN ASSISTANT Pauline Clarke
SENIOR MANAGING EDITOR Mary-Clare Jerram
MANAGING ART EDITOR Amanda Lunn
PRODUCTION CONTROLLER Michelle Thomas

First American Edition, 1997
First American Paperback Edition, 2006
06 07 08 09 10 9 8 7 6 5 4 3 2 1
Published in the United States by
DK Publishing, Inc., 375 Hudson Street
New York, New York 10014

Copyright © 1997 Dorling Kindersley Limited, London
Text copyright © 1997 Nitya Lacroix

All rights reserved under International and Pan-American
Copyright Conventions. No part of this publication may be
reproduced, stored in a retrieval system, or transmitted in any
form or by any means, electronic, mechanical, photocopying,
recording, or otherwise, without the prior written permission of
the copyright owner. Published in Great Britain by Dorling
Kindersley Limited.

Lacroix, Nitya.
    The art of Tantric sex/by Nitya Lacroix.
        p. cm.
    Includes index.
ISBN 0-7566-1877-0
1. Sex instruction. 2. Tantrism. 3. Sex customs – India.
I. Title.
HQ64.L24 1996
613.9'6–DC20   96-33597
                                                         CIP

Text film output by R&B Creative Services,
Great Britain
Reproduced by Colourscan, Singapore
Printing in China by Toppan Printing Co.

See our complete product line at
www.dk.com

CONTENTS

INTRODUCTION

CREATING A SACRED SPACE 18

THE WONDER OF THE BODY 30

GATEWAY TO ECSTASY 50

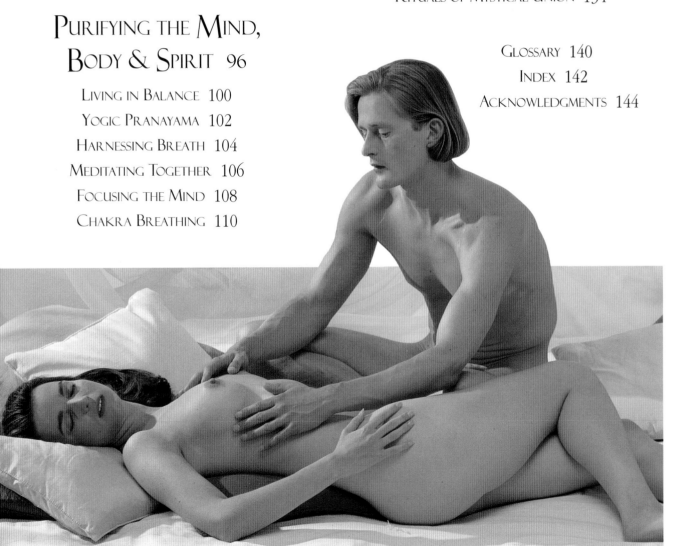

What is Tantric Sexuality?

Tantric Sexuality is Derived From the ancient Indian spiritual philosophy of Tantra, some aspects of which are strikingly pertinent to the modern couple. Throughout the ages, sexuality has been either repressed or exploited. Puritans have decreed that its sole purpose is procreation, while hedonists have utilized it for physical gratification. In recent decades, there has been a welcome debate on sexual issues, but this has focused mainly on enhanced performance techniques for men or on the attainment of better orgasms for women. Tantra decrees that sensual joy is to be celebrated, but it is not the end purpose of sex. It is a means through which you can gain a profound realization of the divine nature of Existence, epitomized in the sexual act.

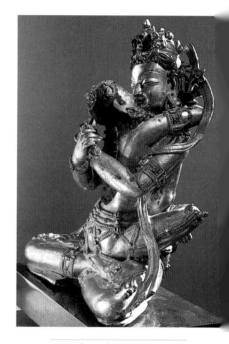

This Tibetan statue depicts ecstatic sexual union as a state of enlightenment.

Tantric Sex *is meditative, spontaneous,*

and intimate lovemaking. Through it you learn to prolong the act of making love and to channel, rather than dissipate, potent orgasmic energies moving through you, thereby raising the level of your consciousness. Tantra transports your sexuality from the plane of doing to the place of being. There is no goal in Tantric sex, only the present moment of perfect and harmonious union. Tantra teaches you to revere your sexual partner and to transform the act of sex into a sacrament of love.

Tantric sex is a journey of body, mind, and soul that enables you to discover a transcendental realm of joy.

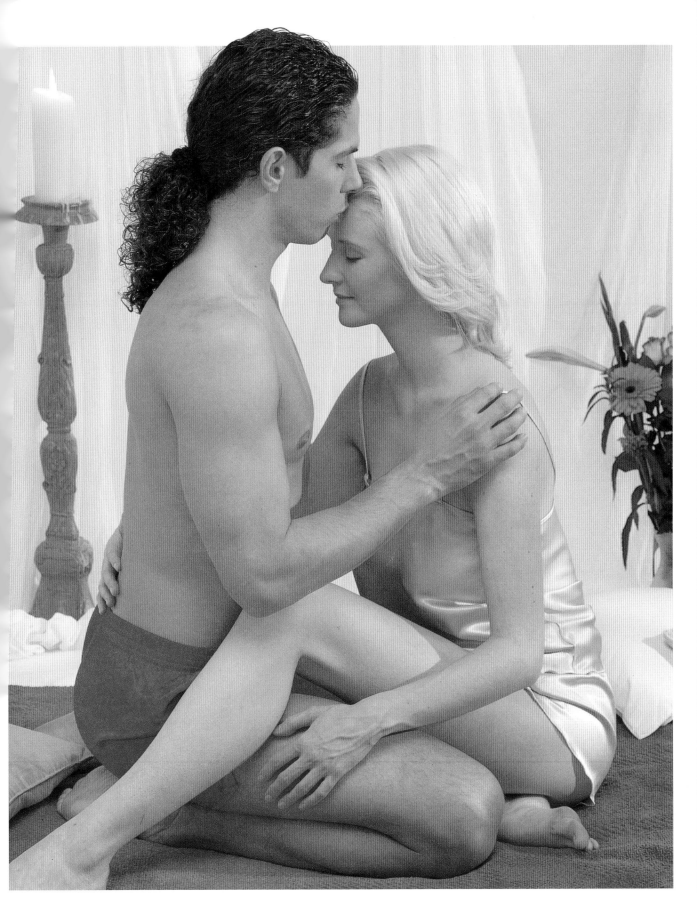

AS A MODERN *couple,* it is not necessary to subscribe to the cultural and spiritual values that originate from traditional Tantric practices. We live in another age, with different lifestyles and belief systems. This book does not go into the depth of practice required by an initiated and committed Tantric disciple. It does, however, adopt aspects of Tantric ritual and weave them together in ways that introduce into your lovemaking a sense of the divine and loving nature of Existence.

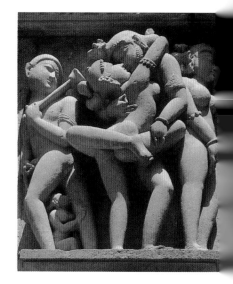

Erotic sculptures adorn the temples of Khajuraho, India, depicting the sacred rites of the sexual mysteries.

TO BRING *a Tantric awareness* into your love-life, it helps to understand its basic concepts. Tantra states that a transcendental quality of consciousness is attained through the merging of dualities into a perfect state of union. Whenever the masculine and feminine principles of energy, which govern all of existence, are in balance, then harmony and equilibrium spontaneously arise. This is the state of Primordial Bliss from which the entire universe was created. According to Tantra, the sexual act is a microcosm of the laws of the universe. It is an enactment of the cosmic principle in which dualities can dissolve into blissful oneness.

TANTRA TEACHES *that lovemaking* between a man and woman, when entered into with awareness, is a gateway to both sexual and spiritual ecstasy. In India, traditional Tantrikas spent many years under the guidance of a spiritual teacher and engaged in elaborate yogic rituals to purify and master the body

Polar principles are brought into harmony through an aware and blissful act of love.

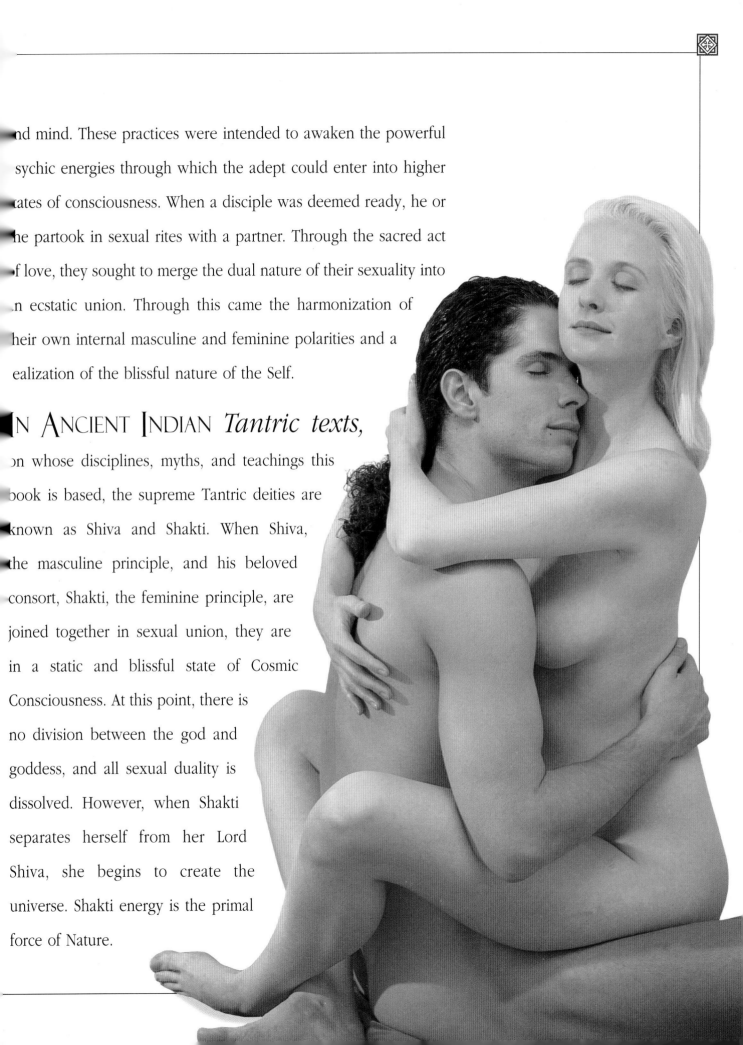

nd mind. These practices were intended to awaken the powerful
sychic energies through which the adept could enter into higher
tates of consciousness. When a disciple was deemed ready, he or
he partook in sexual rites with a partner. Through the sacred act
f love, they sought to merge the dual nature of their sexuality into
n ecstatic union. Through this came the harmonization of
heir own internal masculine and feminine polarities and a
ealization of the blissful nature of the Self.

N ANCIENT INDIAN *Tantric texts,*
on whose disciplines, myths, and teachings this
book is based, the supreme Tantric deities are
known as Shiva and Shakti. When Shiva,
the masculine principle, and his beloved
consort, Shakti, the feminine principle, are
joined together in sexual union, they are
in a static and blissful state of Cosmic
Consciousness. At this point, there is
no division between the god and
goddess, and all sexual duality is
dissolved. However, when Shakti
separates herself from her Lord
Shiva, she begins to create the
universe. Shakti energy is the primal
force of Nature.

EVERY MAN *is the embodiment* of Shiva, and every woman is a manifestation of Shakti. In Tantric temples throughout India, icons abound symbolizing the harmony of sacred sexual union. The most prevalent and significant of these is the lingam and yoni, often carved from wood or stone, which are found in the inner sanctuaries of temples, or even `in simply constructed shrines nestled by a roadside. The lingam represents the hallowed phallus of Shiva and is placed within the divine yoni, which represents the vulva of Shakti.

FEMININE ENERGY *is revered* and honored in Tantra as the catalyst for sexual and spiritual transformation. According to Tantra, the woman is the embodiment of Shakti power, and it is through her that the male Tantric disciple is able to transcend his ordinary human condition to attain sexual ecstasy and spiritual realization. In Hindu Tantra, the woman is perceived as the active principle, the kinetic mover of cosmic energy.

TANTRA ALSO *teaches* a man to honor a woman's sexuality, and to surrender himself to its limitless power. In Tantric lovemaking there is no place for either partner to be selfish. The man, especially, is encouraged to prolong lovemaking and to retain his semen, and to participate in lovemaking sensually and sensitively so that the woman reaches to the heights of her sexual

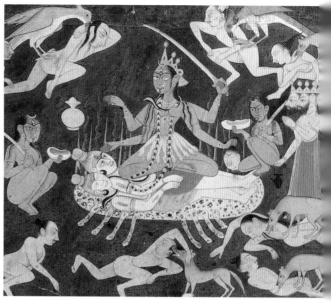

The goddess Kali, in all her terrible glory, is seated in intercourse on the inert and recumbent body of Shiva.

In Tantra, a man must learn to be unafraid of his woman's potent capacity for sexual ecstasy: her Kali aspect.

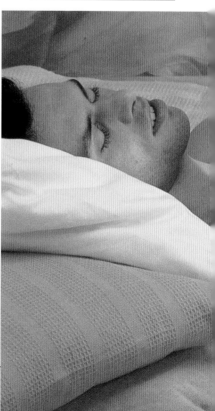

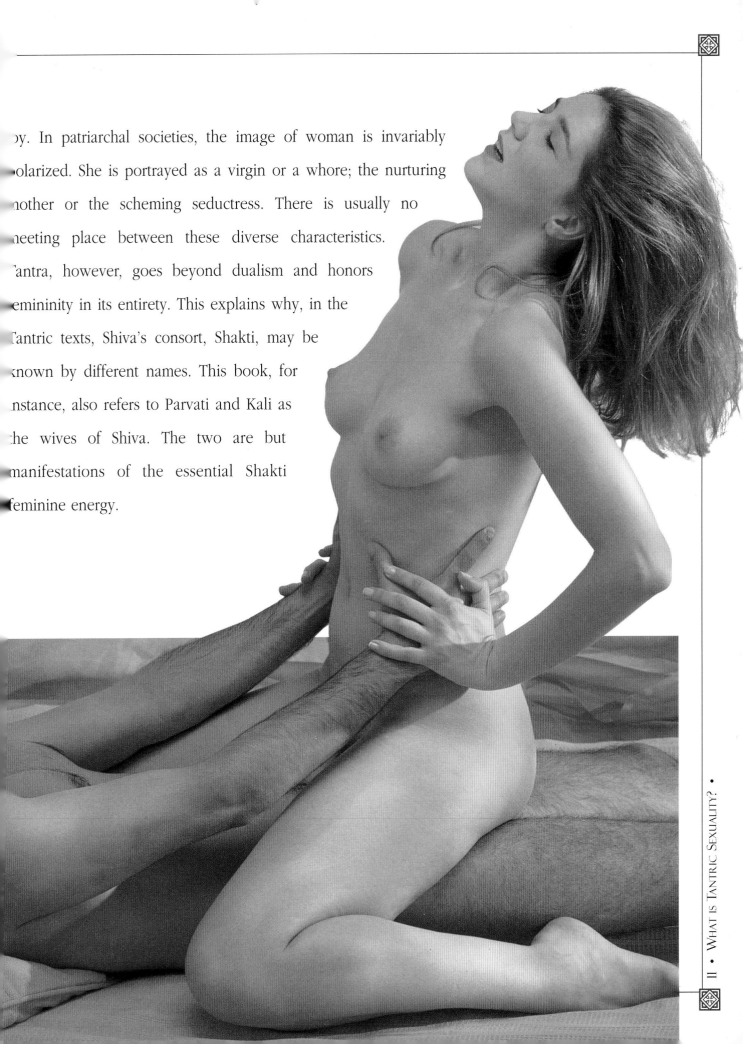

by. In patriarchal societies, the image of woman is invariably polarized. She is portrayed as a virgin or a whore; the nurturing mother or the scheming seductress. There is usually no meeting place between these diverse characteristics. Tantra, however, goes beyond dualism and honors femininity in its entirety. This explains why, in the Tantric texts, Shiva's consort, Shakti, may be known by different names. This book, for instance, also refers to Parvati and Kali as the wives of Shiva. The two are but manifestations of the essential Shakti feminine energy.

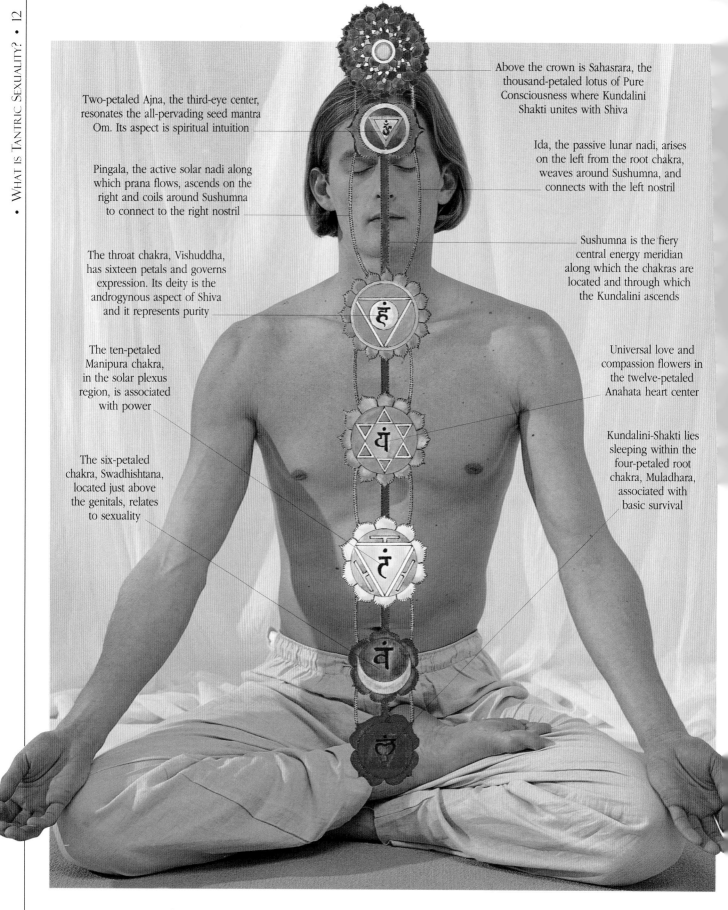

Above the crown is Sahasrara, the thousand-petaled lotus of Pure Consciousness where Kundalini Shakti unites with Shiva

Two-petaled Ajna, the third-eye center, resonates the all-pervading seed mantra Om. Its aspect is spiritual intuition

Ida, the passive lunar nadi, arises on the left from the root chakra, weaves around Sushumna, and connects with the left nostril

Pingala, the active solar nadi along which prana flows, ascends on the right and coils around Sushumna to connect to the right nostril

Sushumna is the fiery central energy meridian along which the chakras are located and through which the Kundalini ascends

The throat chakra, Vishuddha, has sixteen petals and governs expression. Its deity is the androgynous aspect of Shiva and it represents purity

The ten-petaled Manipura chakra, in the solar plexus region, is associated with power

Universal love and compassion flowers in the twelve-petaled Anahata heart center

Kundalini-Shakti lies sleeping within the four-petaled root chakra, Muladhara, associated with basic survival

The six-petaled chakra, Swadhishtana, located just above the genitals, relates to sexuality

ENERGY CENTERS

The seven chakras, located along the Sushumna, are the junction points between the dynamic cosmic plane of existence and the etheric level of the body. These psychic energy centers are windows to the mysteries of the universe, which can be opened by practicing chakra breathing (*see p.110*).

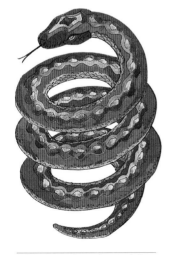

The unawakened Kundalini is represented by a serpent coiled three and a half times at the base of the spine.

PARVATI, *to whom* Shiva revealed the secrets of Tantra, is revered equally as an austere meditator, a lustful wife, and a devoted partner. Kali, as the consort of Shiva, is seen as both a compassionate and a terrifying deity. She is the goddess of Time, presiding over the forces of creation, preservation, and destruction. A dark and awesome persona, she is much worshiped in traditional Tantra as a powerful symbol of womanhood.

TANTRA TEACHES *that the same potent* energies that govern the cosmos exist within the human body. The energy body, though not anatomically discernible, runs parallel, on an etheric level, to the physical body. The energy circuits, or meridians, are called nadis. Three nadis are particularly important: the Sushumna, the central energy channel that corresponds to the spinal column, and the Ida, and Pingala, which intertwine around the Sushumna. Each of the seven main energy centers, called chakras, is represented as a sacred lotus flower. The number of petals on the flower denotes the frequency at which each psychic energy wheel whirls around. On every petal is inscribed a letter of the Sanskrit alphabet, which creates a specific cosmic vibration or sound, known as a mantra.

KUNDALINI *is the raw energy of Shakti.* This dormant force must be awakened if the Tantrika is to achieve enlightenment. Although strict Kundalini yoga is practiced only under the guidance of an enlightened teacher, it is helpful for modern couples to know the Tantric concepts of the subtle body and to become increasingly sensitive to its presence. As consciousness is raised, the Kundalini Shakti ascends through the Sushumna, unlocking the cosmic energies within each lotus center until she reaches her absolute fulfillment in the crown chakra. Only when the Tantrika has raised his or her consciousness to this level can true spiritual enlightenment be achieved.

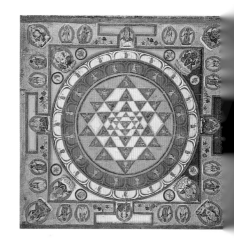

The Shri Yantra represents the creative force of Shakti energy moving out from the still point of Pure Consciousness.

RITUAL *is one of the most important*

ingredients of a Tantric lifestyle. Throughout this book, you are encouraged to participate in the programs and, ultimately, the Tantric lovemaking, in a ritualized manner. This is to help you to endow each event with special significance and, in doing so, to transform both the deed and yourself. Ritual acts encourage you to make a clear intention of becoming more sensitive, aware, and loving – toward your partner and the whole of existence. They elevate the mundane into the spiritual realm. However, within the traditional framework of any ritual, always allow yourself room to be spontaneous and inventive, albeit while remaining intuitively aware, conscious of your breathing, and focused on the spiritual purpose of your Tantric ritual.

IN TRADITIONAL *Tantric worship,* elaborate

rituals, employing mystical aids such as mantras and yantras, formed the basis of all spiritual ceremonies. A mantra is a cosmic sound vibration. By the correct repetition and intonation of a antra, a disciple invokes the energetic resonance of a chosen

eity. A yantra, usually inscribed on paper or metal, is a purely

eometric representation of the manifest form of a cosmic sound

bration, usually symbolizing the body of a Tantric deity. Disciples

se mantras and yantras during Tantric rituals to focus the mind,

duce an elevated state of consciousness, and to invite the

piritual presence of the object of worship to enter into the

eremony. Other Tantric "tools," such as candles, bowls, bells,

hells, and fruit, have a more symbolic ritual function (*see p.26*).

Create a mandala – a circular formation symbolizing the cosmos – using flowers and candles.

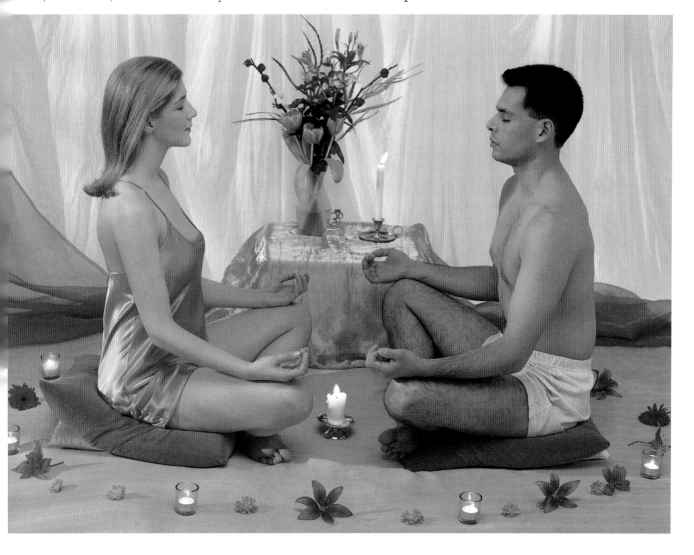

TANTRIC DISCIPLES *participated in rites* of sexual union, known as maithuna, only when they reached a high level of initiation and spiritual awareness, and Tantric texts refer to conjugal union only in the highest terms of reverence. Sexuality, according to Tantra, implies conscious action and shared responsibility if it is to be physically and spiritually meaningful. Never has this precept been more true than it is today.

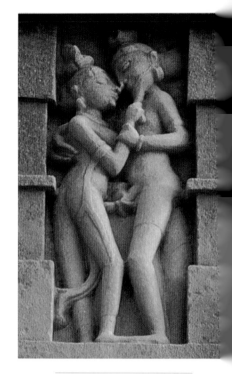

This Khajuraho temple sculpture shows a Tantric couple making love with respect and reverence.

IN TRADITIONAL *Tantric sex rites,* it was not essential for sexual partners to be in established relationships. However, in a modern context, with the advent of the HIV/AIDS virus and other sexually transmitted diseases, Tantric lovemaking functions best within a committed relationship. Tantric texts often refer to the mixing of body fluids, which it calls nectar or love juices, as a potent means of harmonizing male and female energies. This quite clearly conflicts with the advice given today for safer sex practices. You must assess your lovemaking situation cautiously. Safer sex practices are recommended for anyone participating in sexual activity, in any circumstance where the health status, or sexual history, of either partner cannot be fully guaranteed. Do not make love without using a condom, or other reliable barrier contraceptive, unless you are absolutely sure it is safe. By just breathing together, making love slowly and meditatively, and merging joyfully together, you can ensure that your lovemaking is imbued with the spirit of Tantra.

Through kissing and caressing, you can learn to develop intimacy while showing regard for your partner's physical and emotional well-being.

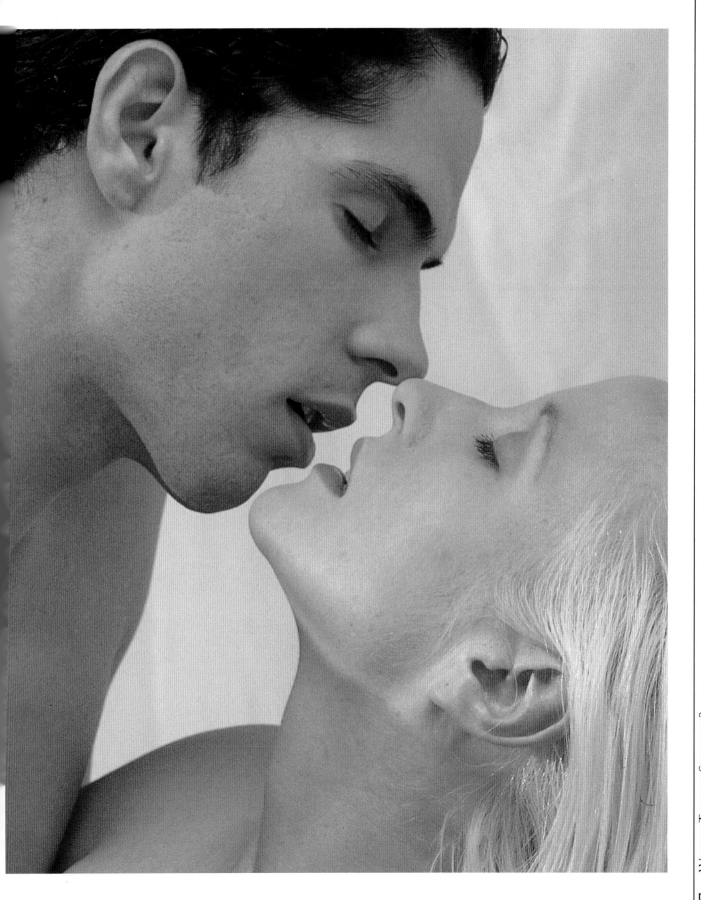

CREATING A SACRED SPACE

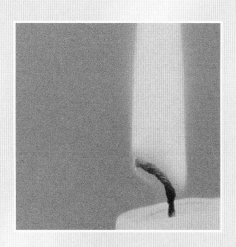

"Decorate the walls of the love-chamber beautifully. Place soft pillows on the bed and liberally sprinkle the sheets with flowers and scent. Burn sweet incense in the room. Then let the man and woman ascend to the throne of love."

ANANGA RANGA

THE SACREDNESS AND PURITY OF THE ENVIRONMENT IN WHICH YOU PERFORM YOUR TANTRIC RITUALS IS very important. Tantra teaches us that the external world of objects

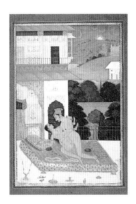

This Indian miniature depicts a Rajput couple making love within their sacred space.

and events and our INTERNAL *realm* of thoughts and feelings are in a constant, interdependent relationship with each other. By creating a harmonious environment, we can establish for ourselves an inner state of TRANQUILITY *and equilibrium.*

IN TRADITIONAL Tantric texts there are precise and detailed instructions on how to set up HALLOWED *places* of worship. Many of these auspicious practices, and the use of Tantric tools, are described in the following pages. However, this chapter is also mindful that as a modern couple, you must CREATE *a sanctuary* within your home that is significant to your own beliefs and lifestyle. The most important aspect of your sacred space is that it is clean, uncluttered, and undisturbed by any outside interference. Ideally, select a room in your home and dedicate it purely to your Tantric rituals. If this is not possible, then allocate a portion of a room to your ceremonies, transforming it into a SACRED *place* through the clever use of materials, rugs, and cushions whenever you need it.

BY USING the same environment continually, you will eventually build up a rarefied and sacred atmosphere within your sanctum. Always dedicate this area to your TANTRIC *ritual* by first lighting a candle and incense, or placing a fragrant flower on your altar. In this way, whether you have created a simple and PEACEFUL *sanctuary* for meditation and yoga or an elaborately sensual ambience for lovemaking, each Tantric ceremony that you perform will be auspicious and deeply meaningful to you and your beloved.

Arrange a sacred space together, filling it with sensual objects.

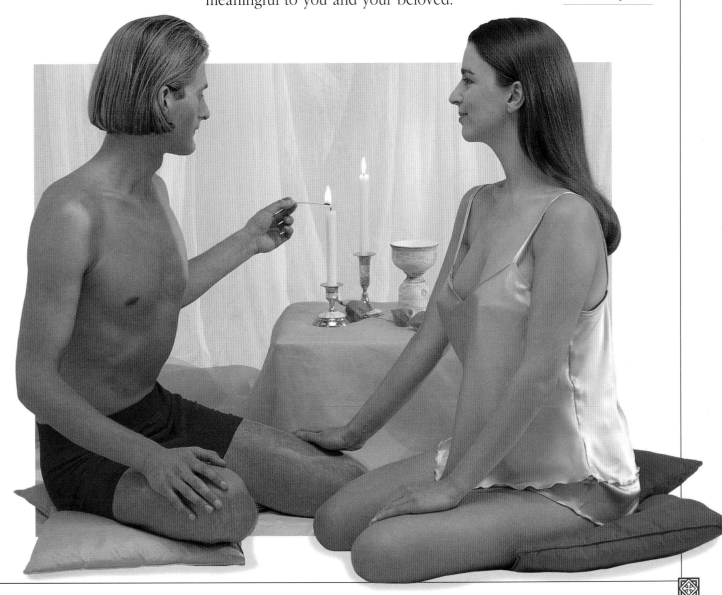

TRANSFORMING YOUR SPACE

THE INGENIOUS USE of materials as drapes and covers, and a luxurious selection of cushions and rugs to spread on the floor, can transform almost any space into a Tantric sanctuary. Even when there is a constraint on actual room space, you can still work wonders with the environment using the right tools and decorative objects. Muslin, traditional Indian saris, and exotic textiles can disguise mundane objects and furniture if it is necessary for them to remain in the room. Introduce into your space the Tantric hues of reds, oranges, purples, terra-cotta, and saffron, which stimulate the chakras, awaken the senses, and ignite sexual energy. A shrine should act as a focal point to remind you that your acts are dedicated to love and consciousness.

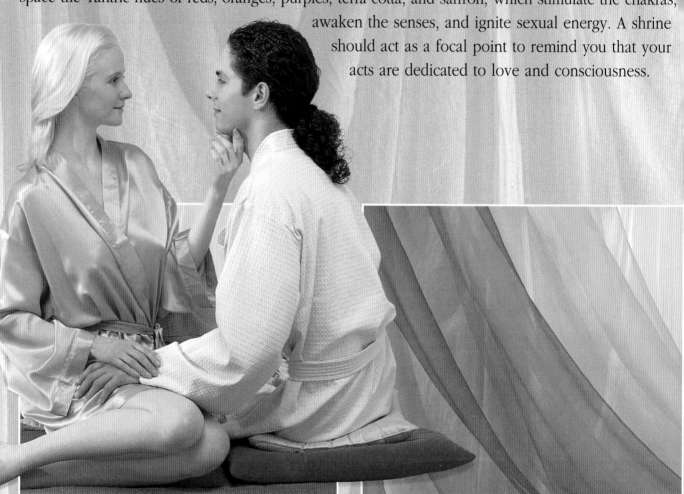

NATURAL FABRICS
Wear clothing made of natural fabric, which is comfortable and sensual to the body. Simple, loose-fitting cotton clothes are ideal for yoga and meditation. Kimonos, which are easy to slip out of, are perfect for times of intimate relaxation.

SENSUAL DRAPES
Hang soft materials around your sanctum to create sensual curving shapes, softening hard corners and adorning plain walls. Chiffon, silk, and muslin drapes can transform the most ordinary room into a billowing temple of love.

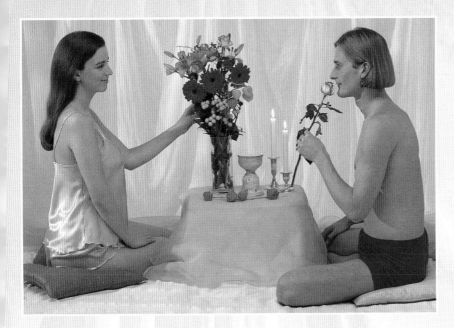

CREATE AN ALTAR

Your Tantric altar can be as simple or as elaborate as you wish to make it, but the objects you place on it should have special meaning and significance to you. Traditional Tantric offerings placed on shrines include incense, ritual foods, and flowers. But only fresh and fragrant flowers are regarded as holy and auspicious in Tantra. A lighted candle should be placed on your shrine during Tantric rituals. As the focal point of much of your meditation, the space in which your shrine is placed will become charged with almost tangible energy. Avoid moving the shrine between rituals.

Adorn your *chamber* with objects upon which the eye *dwells with delight.*" ANANGA RANGA

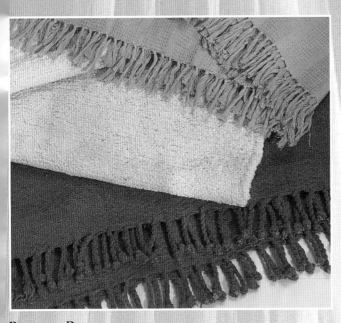

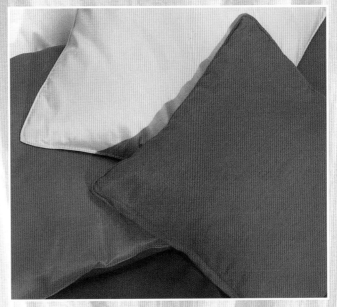

RITUAL RUGS

Lay rugs and sheets of natural fibers over a mattress or directly onto the floor to create the base that will become your bed of love. Tantric texts recommend that lovemaking should take place on beds that are close to the ground.

CUSHIONS FOR COMFORT

Spread cushions around your sanctuary to recline upon and to enhance the sense of comfort and luxury. Choose them in colors that create a Tantric atmosphere. Reserve items such as these solely for the purpose of your Tantric rituals.

SACRED AMBIENCE

DURING ANCIENT TANTRIC CEREMONIES, disciples used incense and perfume in abundance to create a sacred ambience in which to meditate and perform their sexual rituals. The texts describe these holy environments as being richly impregnated with the aromas of camphor, musk, aloe, sandalwood, and other perfumes burned as offerings to the deities. The female disciple was bathed and anointed with a variety of fragrant pastes and oils, such as sandalwood and jasmine, before being worshiped as the Shakti by her sexual and spiritual partner. Tantric rituals were illuminated by moonlight, the warm glow of the flames of fires, or by the pure violet sheen issuing from castor-oil lamps.

OIL RECIPE

In addition to traditional Tantric perfumes, there are alternative aromatic recipes that are both sensual and uplifting. In your essential-oil burner, place 3 drops of frankincense for the elevation of the spirit, 2 drops of cedarwood for spiritual and physical openness, and 2 drops of rose absolute for increasing loving and romantic feelings.

OM SYMBOL

Place a sacred item, which is of special spiritual relevance to you, on a shrine in your sanctum. Tantrikas and traditional Hindus revere the Om symbol, which represents the all-encompassing vibration of universal creation.

OILS TO ANOINT

Learn about the use of aromatic essential oils and discover which of their properties will enhance your Tantric rituals. For anointing and massage, blend the essences with vegetable oils according to instruction and store in beautiful colored bottles.

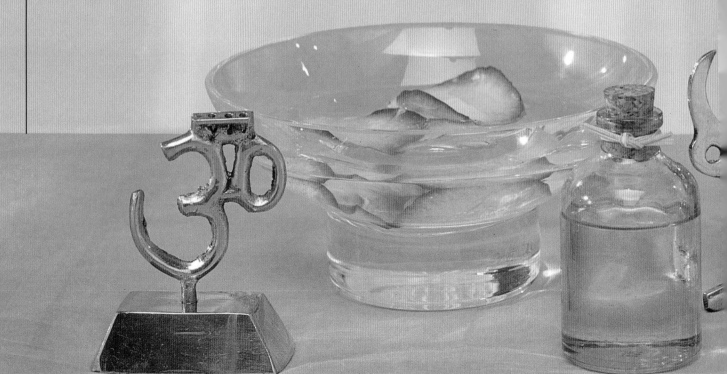

Sprinkle the sheets with
flowers and scents..." ANANGA RANGA

AROUSING AROMA

Smell is the sense of the root chakra, the Muladhara, in which resides the dormant sexual energy of the sleeping Kundalini. Employ aromatic burners to release fragrant scents into your sacred sanctum to stimulate the arousal of sexual energy.

CANDLELIGHT

Bathe your sanctuary in the soft glow of candlelight to create a sensual and spiritually uplifting environment. The flickering shadows cast by the flames add an aura of softness and mystery to your sacred space. Place the candles in ornate but sturdy candle holders.

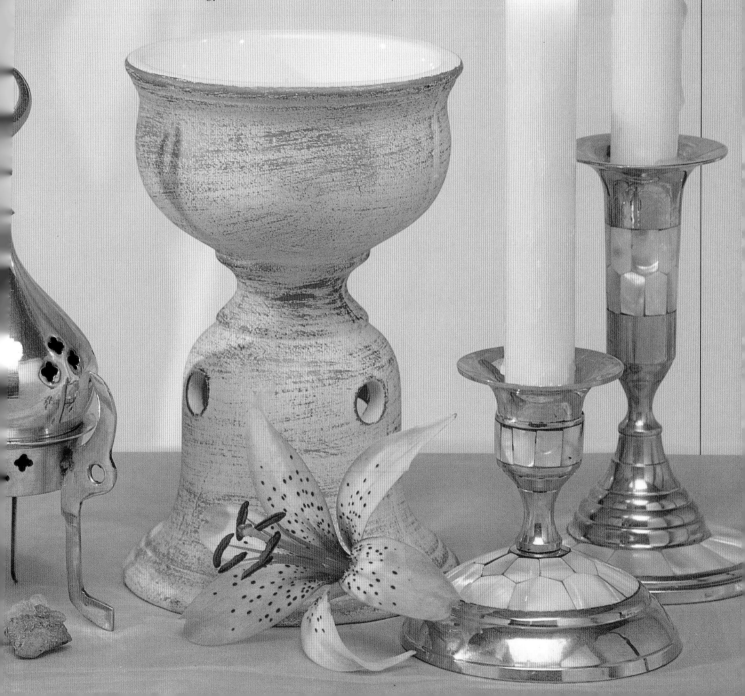

RITUAL OBJECTS

RITUAL OFFERINGS formed the basis of all Tantric worship. Flowers, incense, cloth, trays of food, and bowls of water or wine were among the items proffered to the invoked deities. While the elaborate practices of traditional Tantra may have no philosophical or religious relevance to your lives, you can enrich your acts of love with ritual ceremonies on which you bestow your own significance. Place your gifts on your altar to invite a higher state of consciousness and the Spirit of Love to enter into your lives. Preparing food and wine, and placing them in special containers, is an act of thanksgiving for the bountiful fruits of Nature. Feeding each other morsels of food is a Tantric gesture in recognition of the Divine within each other.

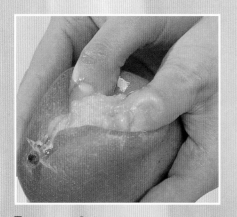 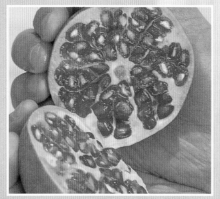 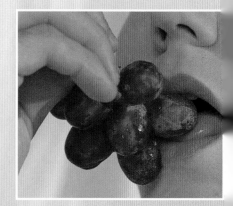

FRUIT OF LIFE

Savor the smells, textures, and tastes of fruits for their sensual qualities, and honor the erotic appearance, which symbolizes the fecundity of Nature. Fruit stimulates the sense of taste associated with the second chakra, situated just above the sex organs.

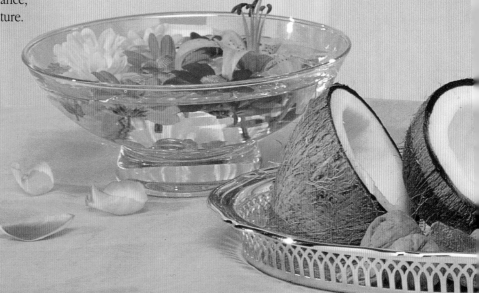

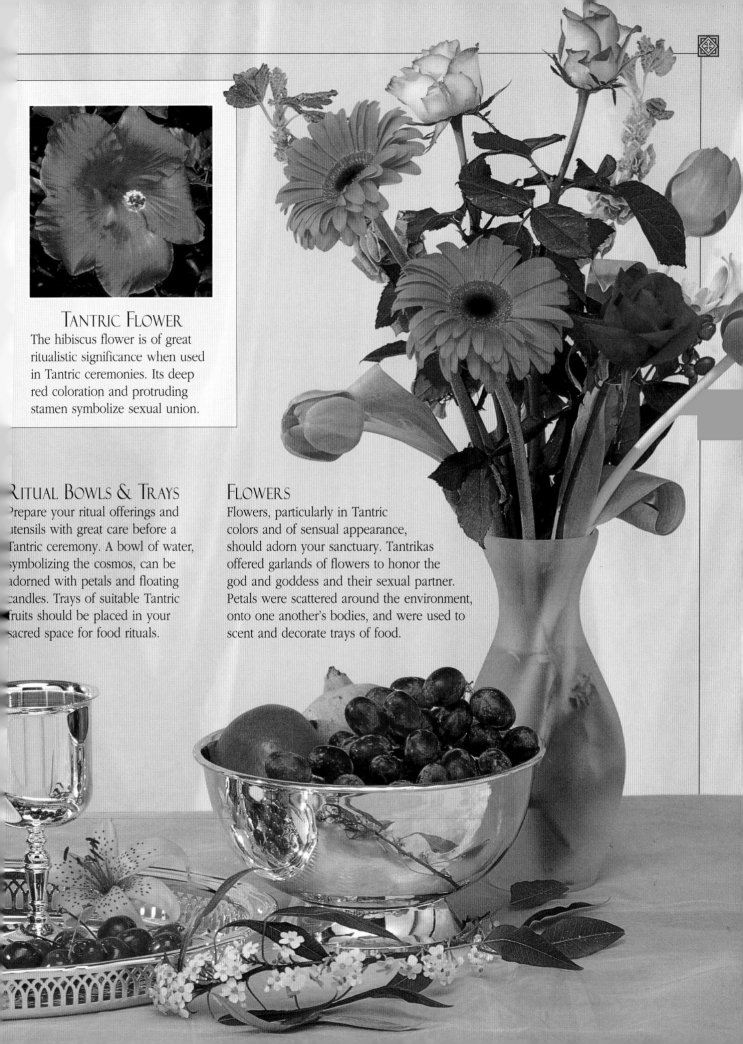

TANTRIC FLOWER

The hibiscus flower is of great ritualistic significance when used in Tantric ceremonies. Its deep red coloration and protruding stamen symbolize sexual union.

RITUAL BOWLS & TRAYS

Prepare your ritual offerings and utensils with great care before a Tantric ceremony. A bowl of water, symbolizing the cosmos, can be adorned with petals and floating candles. Trays of suitable Tantric fruits should be placed in your sacred space for food rituals.

FLOWERS

Flowers, particularly in Tantric colors and of sensual appearance, should adorn your sanctuary. Tantrikas offered garlands of flowers to honor the god and goddess and their sexual partner. Petals were scattered around the environment, onto one another's bodies, and were used to scent and decorate trays of food.

THE COSMIC PLAY

THERE CAN BE NO more sacred an environment in which to meditate and make love than when you are with your beloved close to the awesome majesty of Nature. Everything that is manifested in Nature, according to Tantra, is born out of the ecstatic sexual union of the Tantric deities, Shiva and Shakti. All of existence gives testimony to the blissful merging of male and female energy. Find peace, joy, and equilibrium within your own relationship by going close to the source of creation to practice your Tantric meditations and love rituals. Lie close together and meditate on the infinite space of the sky. Dissolve sexually into one another as the waves dissolve into the immensity of the ocean. All the secrets of Tantra were revealed by Shiva to his beloved wife as they made love high up in the beautiful Himalayan mountains. Let the mysteries of Nature reveal themselves to you.

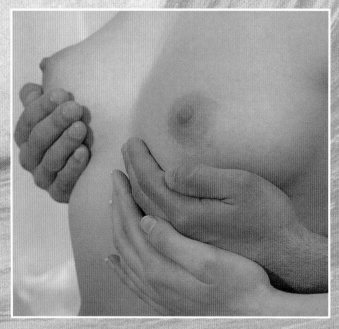
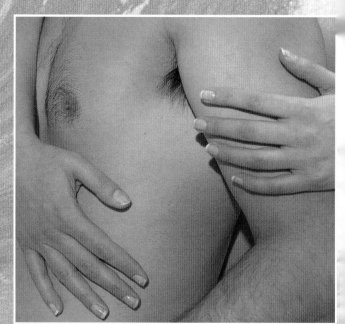

MAKING LOVE IN NATURE

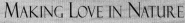

Commit yourselves to taking time off from your daily routines. Go together to a place surrounded by the beauty of nature. Make love close to an ocean where you can hear the sound of the waves; walk hand in hand in a forest; contemplate the vastness of the sky at night.

SEXUAL SYMBOLS IN NATURE

Look for natural objects that can become Tantric yantras of significance for you and your beloved, and place them in your sacred space during Tantric rituals at home. The erotically suggestive appearance of a piece of wood, a shell, or a stone may symbolize to you the principles of the sacred lingam and yoni. Shown here are two natural objects that represent the sacred lingam and yoni. The stone is shaped as an obvious phallic symbol. The magnificent conch shell, with its hollow form and pale pink coloration, corresponds to the vagina and labia of the female genitalia. The conch shell is often associated with Tantric deities.

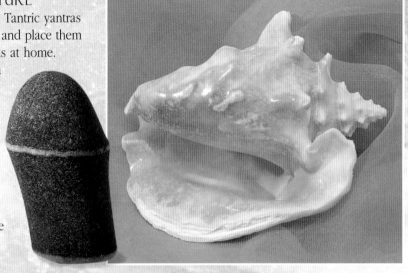

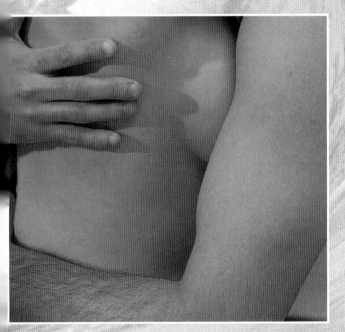

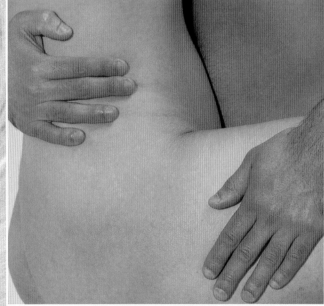

"The *whole universe* is created by the *Shakti* of Shiva." SHIVA PURANA

THE WONDER OF THE BODY

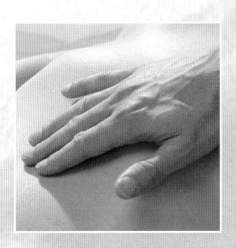

*"He who realizes the
truth of the body can
then come to know the
truth of the universe"*

RATNASARA

IN TANTRIC PHILOSOPHY THE BODY AND THE SPIRIT ARE NOT SEPARATE ENTITIES, NOR IS ONE ELEVATED

above the other. A follower of Tantra learns to love his or her

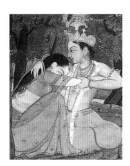

Hindu love gods Krishna and Rhada are often depicted frolicking together.

body, and to awaken its senses to the full. The human body has an enormous capacity for pleasure, and Tantra invites you to celebrate the sensual REALM *of joy*. The awareness gained by this experience can then become a vehicle for transformation in your life. Tantra teaches that within your body reside the same psychic forces that govern the whole of existence. The body is a microcosm of the COSMIC *whole.* Only through the conscious experience of your body's vital energies can you approach the truth of these cosmic mysteries.

TO TRANSFORM YOUR LOVE into the Tantric ideal, you must learn to become increasingly receptive to your own body. Then you will truly be able to become more loving toward your partner's body. This chapter takes you step-by-step through a body-awakening program. It introduces you to the basic key of all Tantric exercises, BREATH *awareness;* it shows you how to accept your body by being more conscious of your judgments; and it teaches you to love and nourish your body with self-care programs, such as touching and anointing.

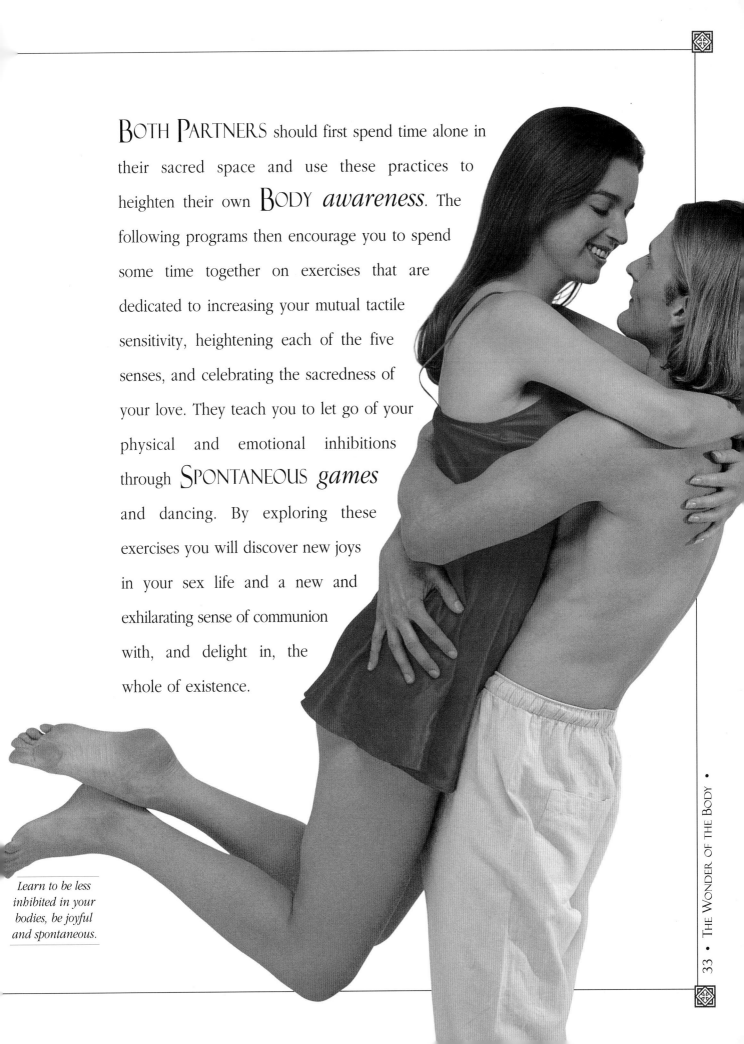

BOTH PARTNERS should first spend time alone in their sacred space and use these practices to heighten their own BODY *awareness*. The following programs then encourage you to spend some time together on exercises that are dedicated to increasing your mutual tactile sensitivity, heightening each of the five senses, and celebrating the sacredness of your love. They teach you to let go of your physical and emotional inhibitions through SPONTANEOUS *games* and dancing. By exploring these exercises you will discover new joys in your sex life and a new and exhilarating sense of communion with, and delight in, the whole of existence.

Learn to be less inhibited in your bodies, be joyful and spontaneous.

BREATH IS LIFE

WHEN WE FOCUS our attention onto our breathing, allowing it to deepen and relax within us, we become more sensitive to our feelings, more alive in our bodies, and more still in our minds. Breath awareness is fundamental to all Tantric disciplines and is employed as a key tool for transformation in yoga, meditation, and lovemaking practices. Breath brings us life and vitality. On inhalation, it oxygenates, nourishes, and energizes our system; on exhalation, it purifies us. Breathing is an automatic function of the body, and yet the majority of people do not breathe fully, using only a fraction of breath's powerful potential. Conscious, regular breathing brings greater harmony and balance to the body and emotions. So spend time each day becoming more aware of your breathing, and you will begin to feel the benefits in all that you do.

RECHARGE YOUR BODY
For 15 minutes each day, use breath awareness to relax your entire body. Lie down comfortably, and consciously direct your breath toward each body part, starting from the toes and moving slowly up to the head. Visualize that each inhalation is revitalizing the area on which you are focusing, and that every exhalation is releasing tension.

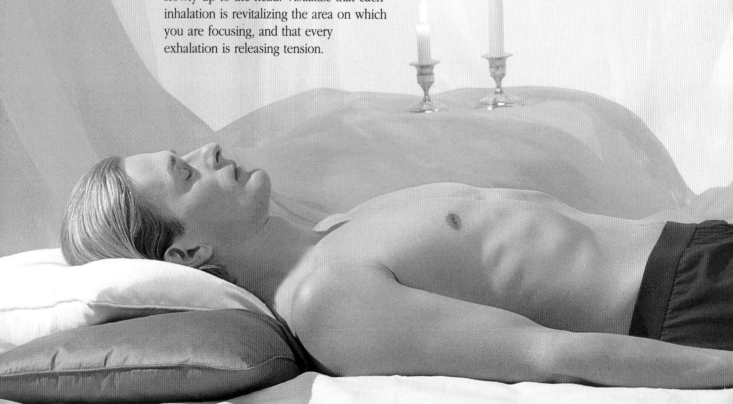

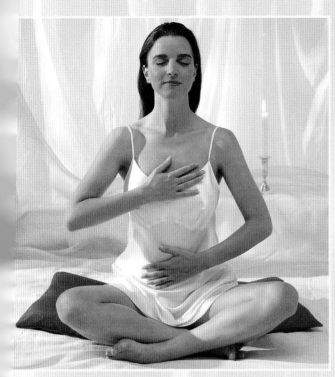

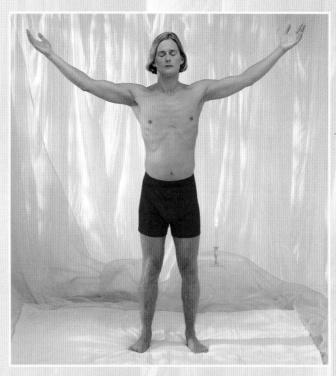

TUNE IN TO YOUR BREATH

Sit comfortably, with a relaxed but lengthened spine, placing your hands over your heart and abdomen. Feel the rise and fall of your breath as you inhale and exhale. Breathe steadily through your nose, allowing the breath to sink deep within.

BREATHING IN MOTION

Feel the vital tremor of physical warmth created by combining breath and movement. Stand with your arms relaxed by your sides. Inhale steadily, raising your arms, palms up, until your fingers touch above your head. Rotate your wrists so that the palms face down, and exhale while lowering your arms until your hands meet in front of you. Repeat 15 times.

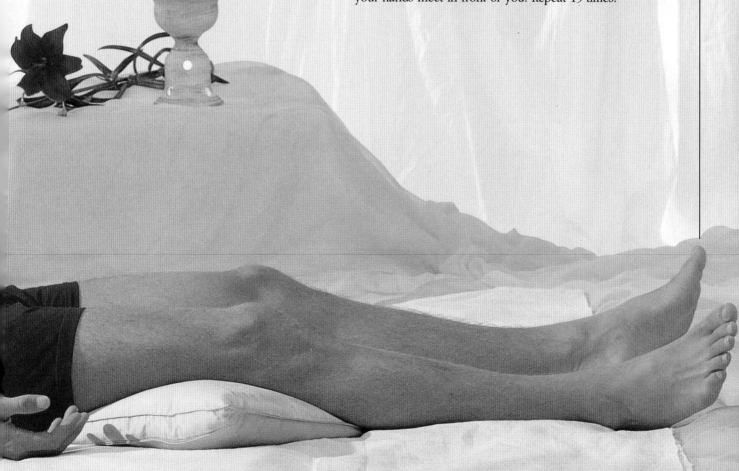

LETTING GO OF JUDGMENTS

TANTRA TEACHES US to honor the body. In the modern world of media images, however, both men and women can be vulnerable to comparing themselves unfavorably with stereotyped "ideals." Negative judgments and comparisons can erode your self-esteem and your ability to love and be loved. Learn to go beyond your judgments, and accept your body in its uniqueness and totality.

RESTORING WHOLENESS ▷

To return a sense of integration to a part of your body, close your eyes and direct your breath and attention toward it. Say to yourself, "I honor this aspect of my body as an intrinsic part of the divine whole."

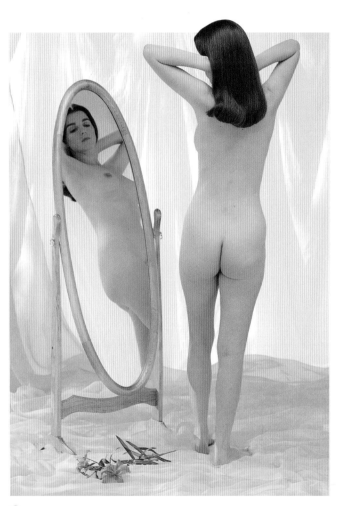

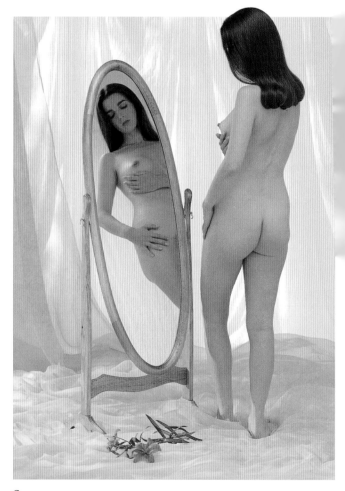

OBSERVATION

Stand naked in front of a full-length mirror and contemplate each aspect of your body, noting objectively, part by part, its physical attributes: color, shape, and muscle tone.

SELF-REFLECTION

Next, be aware of all your judgments and then take note of any associated feelings that arise. Acknowledge all of these thoughts and then consciously let them go.

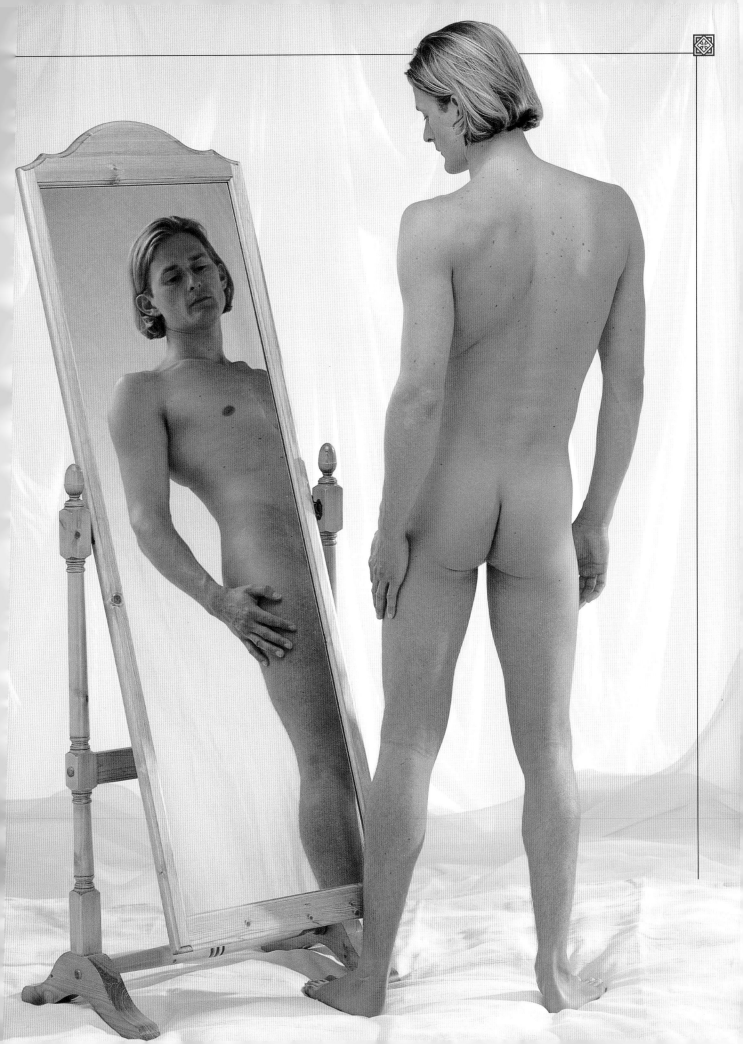

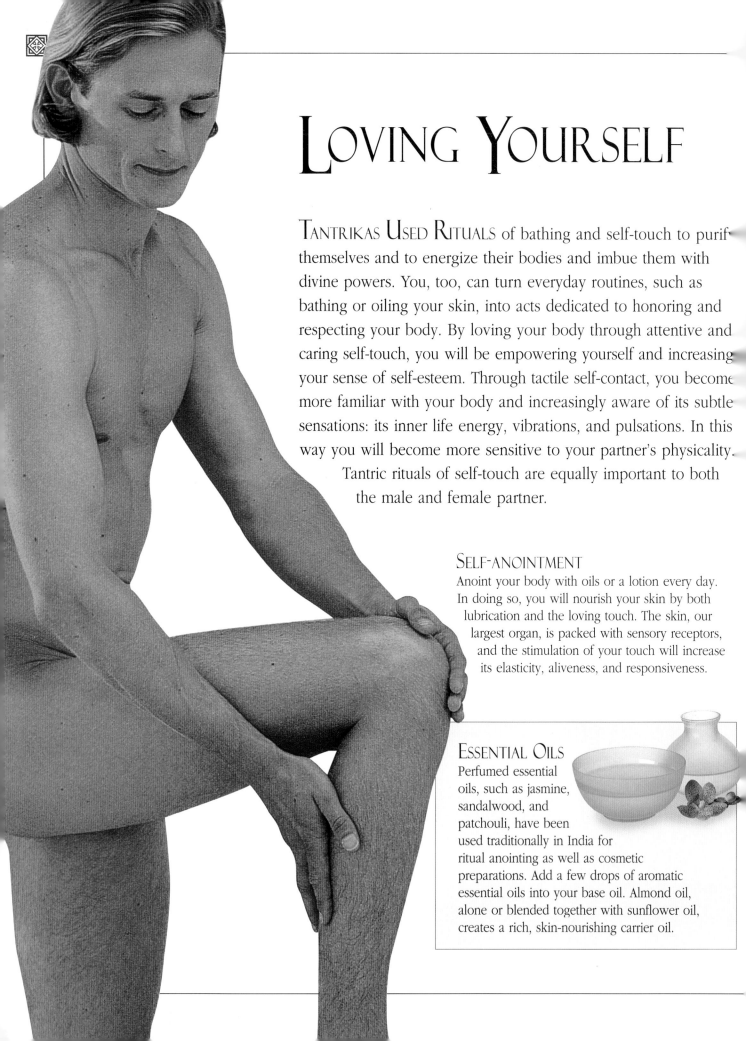

LOVING YOURSELF

TANTRIKAS USED RITUALS of bathing and self-touch to purify themselves and to energize their bodies and imbue them with divine powers. You, too, can turn everyday routines, such as bathing or oiling your skin, into acts dedicated to honoring and respecting your body. By loving your body through attentive and caring self-touch, you will be empowering yourself and increasing your sense of self-esteem. Through tactile self-contact, you become more familiar with your body and increasingly aware of its subtle sensations: its inner life energy, vibrations, and pulsations. In this way you will become more sensitive to your partner's physicality.

Tantric rituals of self-touch are equally important to both the male and female partner.

SELF-ANOINTMENT
Anoint your body with oils or a lotion every day. In doing so, you will nourish your skin by both lubrication and the loving touch. The skin, our largest organ, is packed with sensory receptors, and the stimulation of your touch will increase its elasticity, aliveness, and responsiveness.

ESSENTIAL OILS
Perfumed essential oils, such as jasmine, sandalwood, and patchouli, have been used traditionally in India for ritual anointing as well as cosmetic preparations. Add a few drops of aromatic essential oils into your base oil. Almond oil, alone or blended together with sunflower oil, creates a rich, skin-nourishing carrier oil.

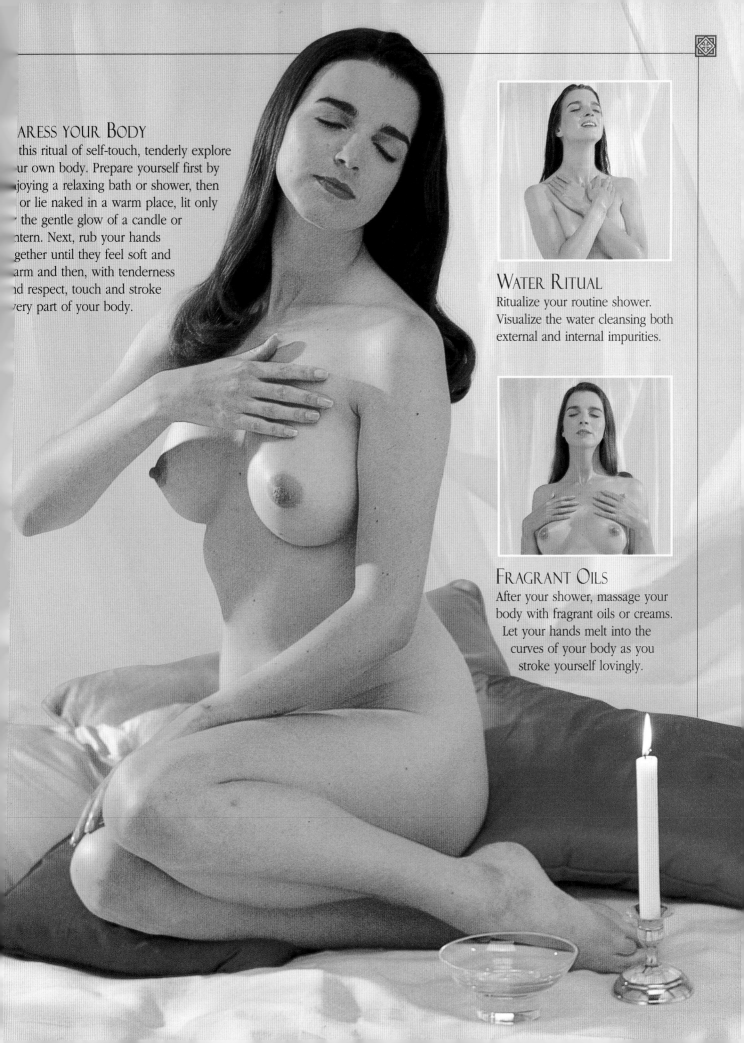

ARESS YOUR BODY

this ritual of self-touch, tenderly explore
ur own body. Prepare yourself first by
joying a relaxing bath or shower, then
or lie naked in a warm place, lit only
the gentle glow of a candle or
ntern. Next, rub your hands
gether until they feel soft and
arm and then, with tenderness
d respect, touch and stroke
very part of your body.

WATER RITUAL

Ritualize your routine shower.
Visualize the water cleansing both
external and internal impurities.

FRAGRANT OILS

After your shower, massage your
body with fragrant oils or creams.
Let your hands melt into the
curves of your body as you
stroke yourself lovingly.

THE TEMPLE

TO A TANTRIC LOVER the human body
is a source of wonder: an endless discovery,
as rich and as mysterious as the cosmos itself.
It is the sacred Temple of the Spirit. Yet we
often know little about our own or our partner's
bodies outside the physical contact of making love.
Once we become adults, it is difficult to regain the
innocent attitude toward the body that was naturally
ours during early childhood. The exploration of touch
described here will help both you and your partner to
rediscover that innocence outside the context of a sexual
situation. This exercise can also help to revive spontaneity
in a sexual relationship that has been dulled by routine.

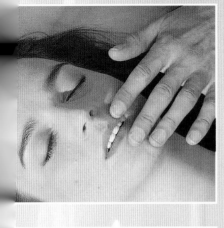
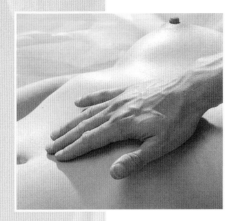
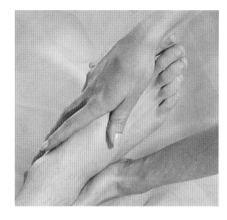
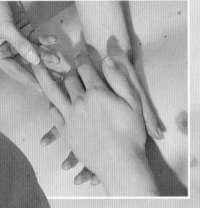
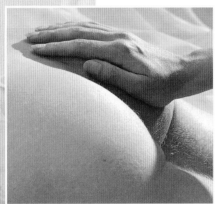
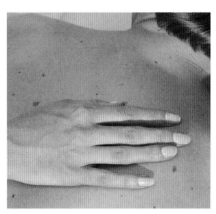

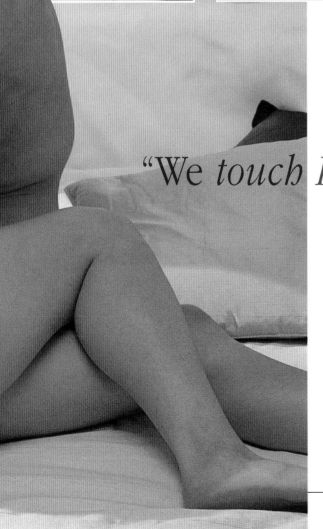

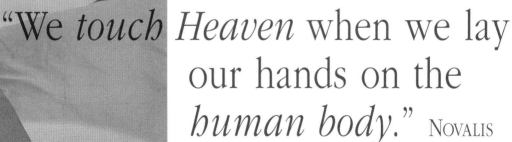

FEEL THE TACTILE SENSATIONS
Touch your lover's body as if for the first time. Become totally absorbed in the tactile sensations of hair, skin, bones, contours, and even body temperature and texture. The receptive partner should focus attention solely on the experience of being touched.

"We *touch Heaven* when we lay our hands on the *human body.*" NOVALIS

BE IN TOUCH WITH YOUR PARTNER'S BODY
Prepare your space to be warm, sensual, and inviting. Decide which partner, on this occasion, will be receptive and which will be active. At another time, the roles should be reversed. For up to an hour, touch, feel, and explore the whole of your partner's body in a loving, respectful, and nonsexual way. Later, discuss your experiences.

HEIGHTENING THE SENSES

THE FIVE SENSES of the physical body – smell, taste, sight, touch, and hearing – link our internal sense of self with the external world of experience. By heightening your senses, you open the doorways to greater sensory perception, joy, and inner transformation. Tantra encourages you to delight in your senses and to relish the pleasures they can bring you. Perform a sensory awakening ritual with your lover in a beautifully prepared room filled with enhancing aids. Choose who, on this occasion, will be the active or passive partner. Dedicate up to 15 minutes to stimulating an individual sense. Rest between each sense ritual to assimilate its particular unique experience.

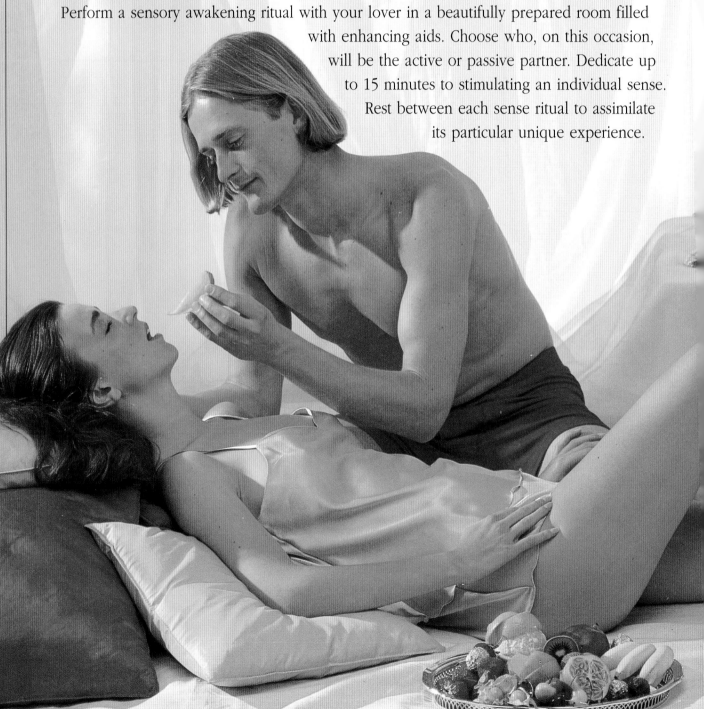

THE SENSE OF SMELL

[Sm]ell is the sense related to the base [ch]akra and to the element of earth. [Pr]epare aromatic blends of essential [oil]s, each capturing a different type of [fra]grance, such as floral, herbal, minty, [mu]sky, or woody. Then offer them, [on]e at a time, for your lover to smell. [As]k your partner to close her eyes so [th]at she can focus exclusively and [in]tensely on the different perfumes. [W]ait for some moments between each [ar]omatic offering, so that she can fully [ap]preciate each olfactory effect. You [ca]n also bring to her the scents of [di]fferent flowers and fruits selected [e]specially for this occasion.

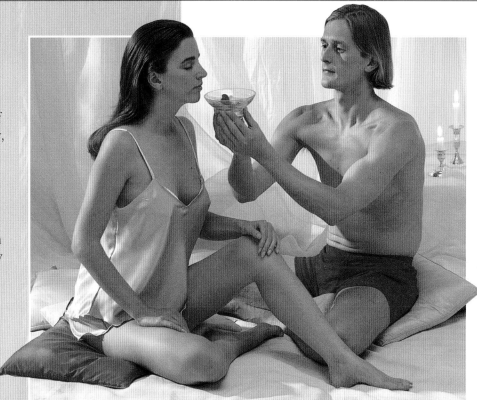

"I am the *vital breath...*" SHIVA PURANA

THE SENSE OF TASTE

Help your lover to heighten her sense of taste by lovingly preparing and serving titbits of food like fruit or chocolate for her to sup and nibble. Ask her to close her eyes so that she can concentrate on tasting each morsel, savoring the full range of succulent, sweet, salty, smooth, and crisp flavors and textures. Taste is the sense of the second chakra and is associated with the element of water.

BALANCING THE ELEMENTS

According to Tantric teachings, each sense is related to a corresponding chakra in the subtle energy body, and each is ruled by one of the five elements: earth, water, fire, air, and space. Tantra teaches that all aspects of life are composed of the five elements, and that harmony exists only when these elements are in balance. By awakening our senses, we can bring greater equilibrium to the elemental forces at work within us. Ancient Tantric texts explain how ecstatic lovemaking generates and balances the five elements within the body. When we make love blissfully, with all of our senses fully engaged, then the elements are harmonized, thus restoring health and vigor to the physical body's vital organs, joy and equilibrium to the mind, and primal bliss to the spirit.

THE SENSE OF SIGHT

Looking is not the same as seeing, just as hearing is not the same as listening. When we look at something, we often miss the finer details of what we observe. Truly seeing involves focusing your whole attention. Enhance the sense of sight by gathering together a visually varied array of objects for your partner to look at. Place before her, one at a time, items such as shells, stones, fabrics, and flowers. Encourage her to focus on them, absorbing the details of their sensual and stimulating shapes, shades, and colors. Then let her gaze at your face, so she can visually absorb its unique character.

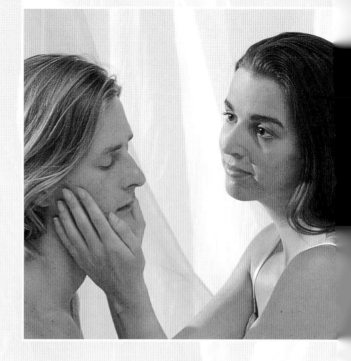

THE SENSE OF TOUCH

Touch brings nourishment to the mind, body, and soul. How we were touched in our infancy helped to establish our self esteem. Through touch, the sense of the skin, we connect our inner reality to the world surrounding us. Heighten your lover's tactile senses, by caressing and blowing lightly onto her skin. Trail soft, sensuous materials, such as silk, chiffon, and lace, over her body. Touch is the sense of the heart chakra and is associated with the element of air.

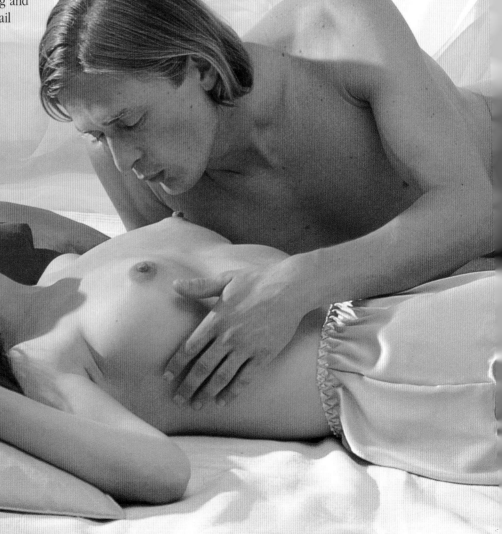

THE SENSE OF SOUND

...come more sensitive to the subtleties of sound. Prepare a ...mber of auditory tools for your partner to hear, including ...lifting excerpts of music, bells, chimes, and easy-on-the-...r musical instruments. Ask your partner to listen attentively ...the natural sounds in the environment. Then softly whisper ...ing words into her ear, hum, and chant. Walking around ...r, introduce her to a whole variety of resonant sounds and ...rations. By closing her eyes, her auditory sense will be intensified. Sound is the sense relating to the throat chakra and its element is space.

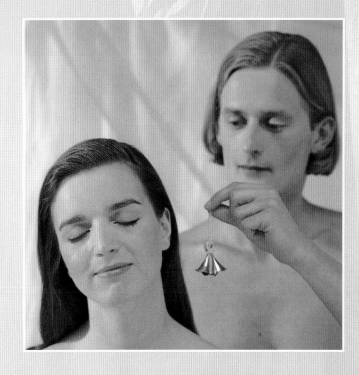

"*O beautiful lady*, the body consists of *five elements*. It arises from them and *merges* in them." SHIVA PURANA

THE CELEBRATIVE BODY

REDISCOVER your childlike sense of fun and spontaneity by finding the time to play games with your lover. Shed the burdens of adult responsibility when you are alone together and free your bodies and minds from the tensions and inhibitions that can restrict your innate vitality. Be naked and innocent with each other, and celebrate the aliveness of your bodies as you roll around together without a care in the world. By delighting in this more abandoned side of yourselves, you will nourish your relationship with humor and joy.

ANIMAL INSTINCTS
Act the animal together. Pretend to be lions roaring at one another. Let the primal sounds reverberate from deep within you. Conclude this ritualistic play by rubbing and nuzzling your naked skin against your lover's body.

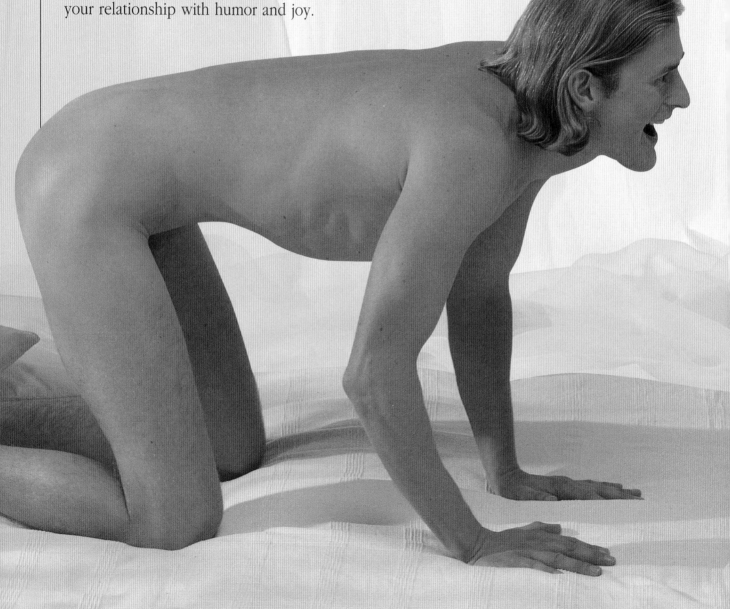

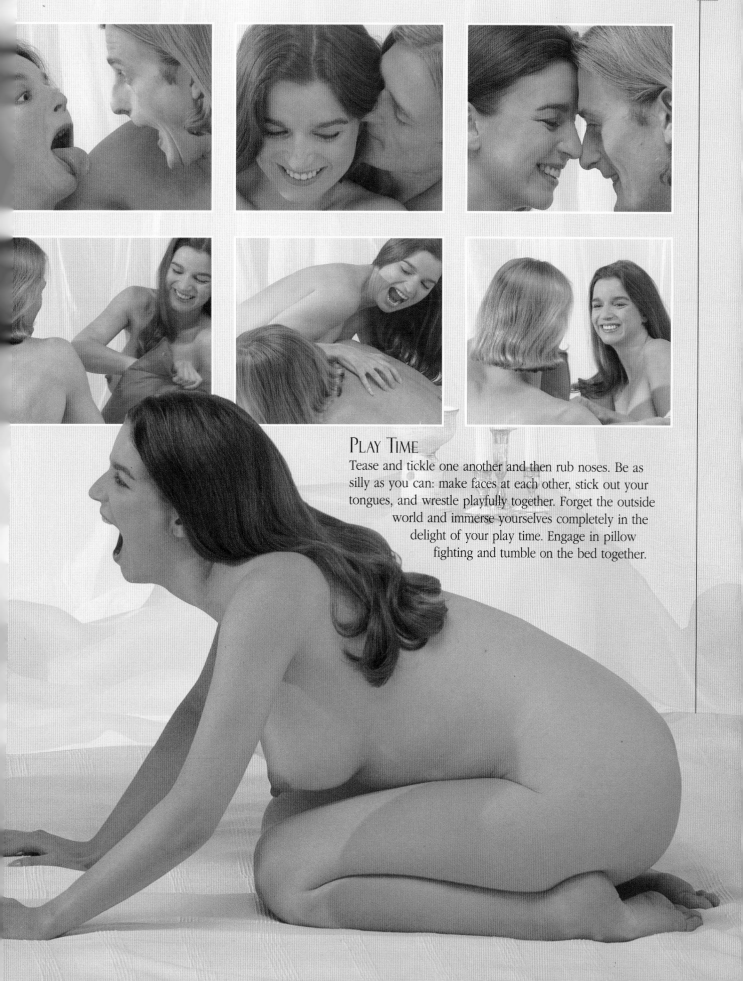

PLAY TIME

Tease and tickle one another and then rub noses. Be as silly as you can: make faces at each other, stick out your tongues, and wrestle playfully together. Forget the outside world and immerse yourselves completely in the delight of your play time. Engage in pillow fighting and tumble on the bed together.

DIVINE DANCE

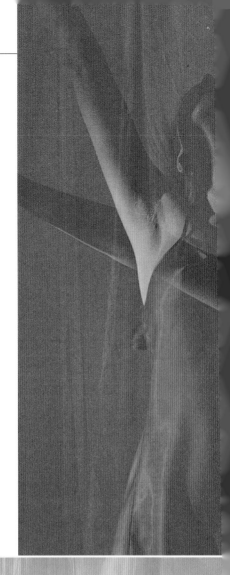

DANCE IS A POWERFUL TOOL for awakening sexual energy, and has always been a part of Tantric ritual. In ancient India, it was the temple dancing girls, known as devadasis, who initiated disciples into the sacred sexual mysteries. By abandoning yourself ecstatically into dance, so that every cell in your body throbs with aliveness, you can transform movement into a transcendental experience. Create an ambience where you can dance without inhibition, alone or with your partner, for up to an hour. Select music that helps to free and inspire you. Bring your body, heart, and soul into the dance. Let the movements arise out of the sheer joy of expressing yourself physically, emotionally, and spiritually. Dissolve into the dance, and let it become a celebration of love and life as if you are dancing with the Divine.

"I am the originator…, abiding in *supreme bliss*. I dance *eternally*."

KURMA PURANA

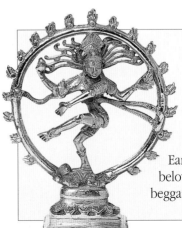

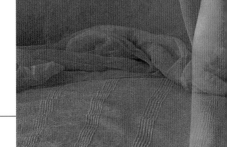

DANCE OF THE SHIVA NATARAJ

The Shiva Nataraj statue depicts the mighty god performing his ecstatic Cosmic Dance, presiding over the never-ending cycle of creation and destruction. Shiva is known as the Lord of the Dance. His dancing filled the Earth and skies. He danced ecstatically with his beloved in the forests of India, and, disguised as a beggar, danced to win the hand of his wife, Parvati.

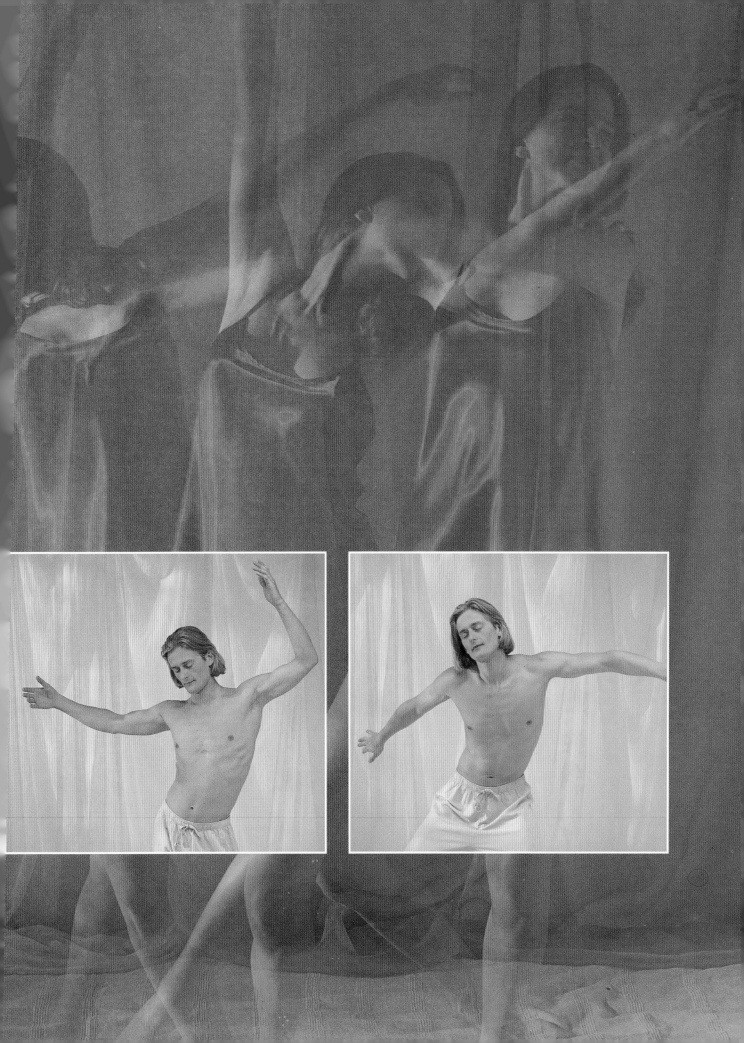

Gateway to Ecstasy

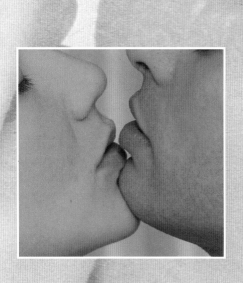

"We two will make love on a
beautiful bed, all strewn with
flowers. I shall take much pleasure
in kissing your bright red lips and
caressing your body."

PADMA PURANA

TANTRIKAS CONSIDER SEXUALITY TO BE THE GATEWAY TO ECSTASY. EVEN IN THE MOST FUNDAMENTAL

way, your relationship contains the potential for cosmic bliss.

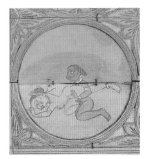

Many Tantric sexual postures imitate animal mating positions. Shown here is the Elephant posture.

Every sexual act between a man and woman is, on some level, an enactment of the meeting of masculine and feminine energies which, on a macrocosmic level, is the basis of UNIVERSAL *harmony*.

When your sexual relationship is at once meditative and stimulating, it becomes an instrument for inner transformation.

TANTRA URGES you to embrace your sexuality wholeheartedly. It does, however, ask that you become more meditative, aware, and loving in your sexual relationship, so that you can find happiness and joy from conjugal union with your partner. This chapter seeks to encourage you and your lover to be OPEN *and honest* about your own sexuality and about your sexual relationship. Even in the most secure partnerships, it can be difficult to talk about sexual issues. Often people do not broach sexual issues even in their own hearts and minds. To open yourself up to the Tantric path, you should spend some time alone in your sacred space, exploring your own sexuality. Discover what turns you on, and SHARE *this knowledge* with your lover.

BEFORE INTRODUCING the more complex concepts of Tantra into your sexual relationship, the exercises on the following pages are designed to make sure that both of you are comfortable, free of guilt, and happy in your normal sex life. Seek to make it HEALTHY *and harmonious*, so that it can become the perfect stepping stone into the mutual exploration of Tantra.

BY FREEING yourselves of inhibitions, you can discover your true SEXUAL *nature.* You will release energies that can rekindle flames of passion doused by taboos, routines, and the pressures of modern living. The woman will discover her natural role as initiatress in Tantric sex. You will both learn to enter more fully, and treasure, each sensual and sexual moment you spend together.

Tantra honors sexuality as an instrument of inner transformation.

THE SACRED GATES

THE FIRST STEP to a higher sexual consciousness is to develop a healthy and respectful attitude toward your own genitals. Tantra regards the sexual organs as sacred parts of the human body. By becoming familiar with these intimate areas, you honor the fundamental abode of your sexuality. Learning to know and love these parts of yourself often entails the sometimes emotionally painful process of overcoming old taboos and guilt complexes. Nevertheless, each partner should take time alone to explore his or her sexual organs. Through breath and visualization, increase your awareness of, and your connection to, these sacred parts of your body.

YONI RITUAL

Use a hand mirror to gaze at your vulva. Note its unique shape and color, and then, parting the outer and inner lips with your fingers, look at your clitoris and vaginal entrance.

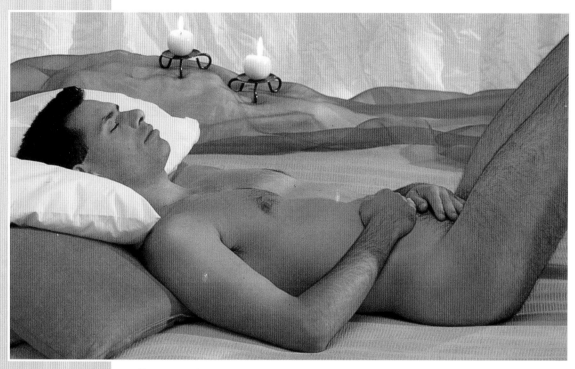

GENITAL RELAXATION

Let go of tension in the pelvic and genital region. Lie down and relax your whole body. Inhale deeply into your abdomen and then imagine the breath is being slowly exhaled through your genitals and anus. Visualize this area becoming warmer and softer with each outgoing breath.

GAIN CONTROL

Deepen your connection to, and your control over, your genital responses by exercising the pelvic floor muscles (*see p.92*), which surround and support your sexual organs. By increasing the flow of blood to the genital area you will not only revitalize, strengthen, and tone the tissues, you will also heighten your sexual responses, while maintaining your control over the buildup of your orgasmic climax. These exercises are of enormous benefit to both partners during Tantric lovemaking.

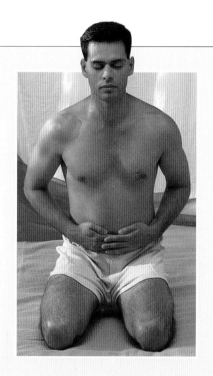

HEALING THE LINGAM & YONI

THROUGH TALKING, touching, and entering into intimate, still union with one another, you can ease away old hurts and negative memories connected to your sexual past. You can create a more positive and respectful attitude toward your sexuality and your sexual organs. This emotional healing of the lingam and yoni (as the sacred penis and vagina are referred to in Sanskrit Tantric texts) will enable you to transform your sexual relationship and will open up a deeper level of trust between you and your lover.

"The *Universe* is in the nature of *male and female.*"

SHIVA PURANA

SHARING ▷

Allocate quality time and take it in turns to talk openly and honestly with each other about your sexual feelings, hopes, and fears. When it is your turn to speak during a session, try to talk candidly for up to 15 minutes. While your partner is talking, listen carefully without interrupting. Be respectful to each other's vulnerability.

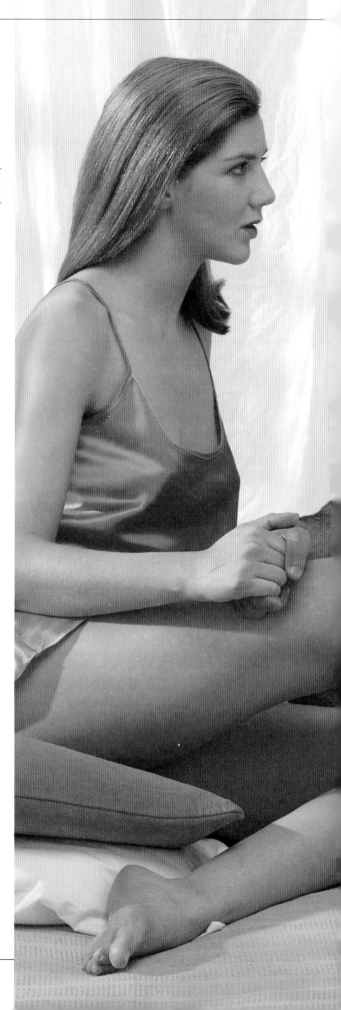

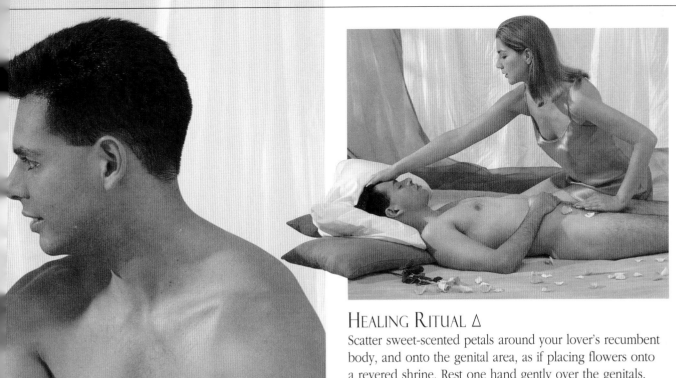

Healing Ritual △

Scatter sweet-scented petals around your lover's recumbent body, and onto the genital area, as if placing flowers onto a revered shrine. Rest one hand gently over the genitals, placing the other hand, for two or three minutes at a time, onto the psychic energy centers such as the abdomen, solar plexus, heart, or forehead. Pour warmth and love into your hands, while your partner relaxes deeply and absorbs your healing and integrating touch. During another session, reverse roles and repeat the healing process.

Uniting the Lingam & Yoni

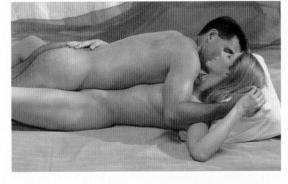

Bring the lingam and yoni together in a tranquil, undemanding, and healing atmosphere of stillness, intimacy, respect, and love. The man should enter the woman's vagina while his penis is relatively soft. Remain relaxed and unmoving, and direct your breath gently toward your genitals. Prolong this ritual for as long as you both feel comfortable, any time that you seek deep communion without active intercourse.

THE LOVER WITHIN

LOOK WITHIN YOURSELF for the wellspring of your sexual ecstasy, for you are the source of your own orgasmic joy. By learning to pleasure your own body, you will discover how and where you like to be touched. By exploring the mysteries of your own unique eroticism, you can then share these treasures with your partner. Whether you are a man or a woman, you will benefit from creating a ritual of sensual self-pleasuring, not only because it increases your tactile sensitivity and your orgasmic potential, but also because it frees you from old taboos about masturbation. Prepare a beautiful sanctuary of love as a setting for this ritual of meeting your inner lover where you have all the undisturbed time that you need.

MALE PLEASURING

Tantra does not encourage a man to ejaculate his semen through masturbation. It is perceived as a waste of his vital life essence. However, self-pleasuring rituals can enhance a man's whole body sensuality if the occasion is treated with an appropriate sense of honor and respect. Bathe and anoint your skin with lotion. Scent your sanctum with oils especially suited to male sexuality, such as jasmine and sandalwood. Arouse your entire being through self-touch.

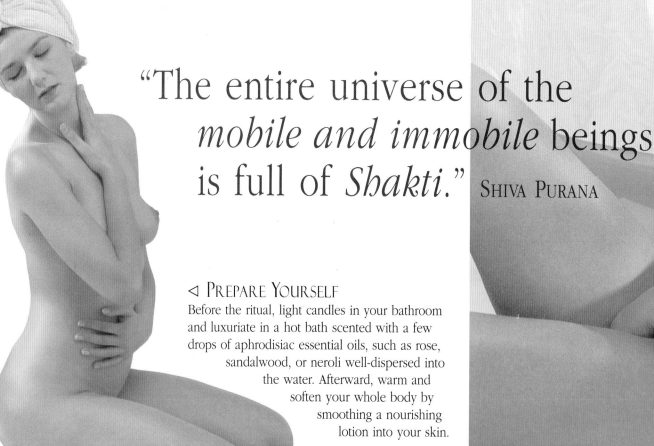

"The entire universe of the *mobile and immobile* beings is full of *Shakti.*" SHIVA PURANA

◁ PREPARE YOURSELF

Before the ritual, light candles in your bathroom and luxuriate in a hot bath scented with a few drops of aphrodisiac essential oils, such as rose, sandalwood, or neroli well-dispersed into the water. Afterward, warm and soften your whole body by smoothing a nourishing lotion into your skin.

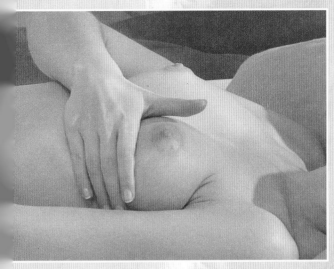

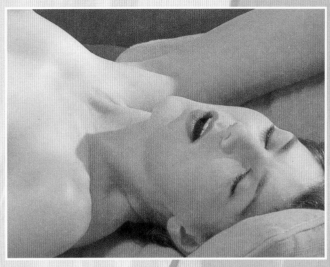

AROUSING TOUCHES

Lying down on your bed, caress your whole body, including your face, breasts, belly, and thighs. Let your fingers explore the soft folds of your labia and sensually stroke your vagina and clitoris in all the ways that bring you great pleasure.

LETTING GO INTO ORGASM

Positive sexual fantasy can initiate and heighten arousal. However, try not to become stuck in cerebral images, but rather submerge yourself deeply in the actual physical experience. Pulsate your pelvic floor muscles to increase orgasmic sensations and when you are filled to the brim, move, sigh, moan, and express your eroticism without inhibition. Surrender your body to the waves of pleasure.

ASSIMILATING PLEASURE

Do not hurry towards orgasm, but take the time to absorb your sexual sensations. As your arousal naturally increases, relax and breathe deeply and steadily, as if drawing the heightening orgasmic wave up through your entire body.

SHARING SEXUAL SECRETS

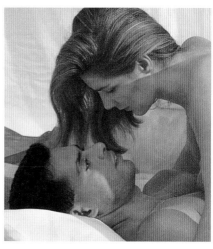

OBSERVE CLOSELY
By watching your lover pleasure himself,
you can learn how to apply the right
degree of manual pressure, rhythm,
and speed when you arouse him.

MOST PEOPLE are able to enter a mental world of sexual
fantasy, the very secrecy of which fuels the fire of its eroticism.
Even within a committed relationship, it is completely reasonable
to want to keep some of your sexual fantasies purely to yourself.
There are times, however, when sharing sexual secrets enriches
your love life. Talking about, and showing each other, exactly
how you like to be touched sexually, will enlighten you both in
the ways in which you can better pleasure your partner. Setting
aside time to explore these issues will increase the intimacy and
trust between you, thus creating a strong foundation for a loving
and enduring Tantric relationship.

"By reciprocal *indulgence*, their *love endures*." KAMA SUTR

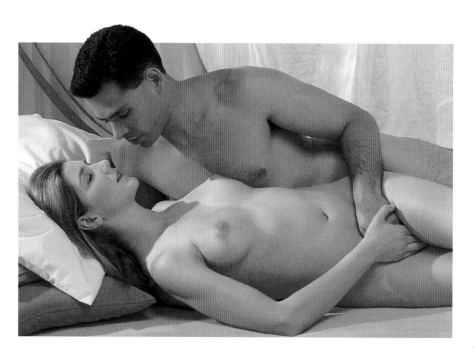

◁ GUIDING HAND
Let your partner guide your hand as she
shows you the varying ways in which
she likes to sexually stimulate herself.
Note, especially, how she guides your
hand to gently caress her labia, and
how she moves and touches her body
as she becomes increasingly aroused.
Be particularly sensitive to when and
how she touches her clitoris, and notice
the rhythm and pressure she applies to
it – especially in the moments before
she reaches her climax.

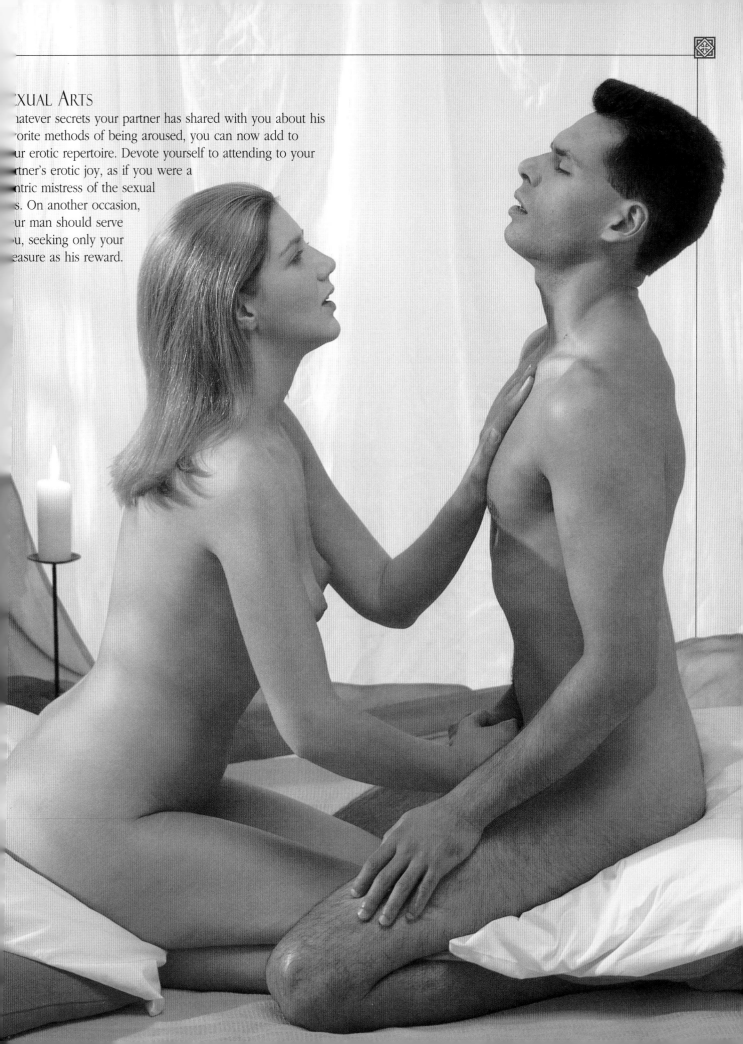

XUAL ARTS

...hatever secrets your partner has shared with you about his
...orite methods of being aroused, you can now add to
...ur erotic repertoire. Devote yourself to attending to your
...rtner's erotic joy, as if you were a
...ntric mistress of the sexual
...s. On another occasion,
...ur man should serve
...u, seeking only your
...easure as his reward.

THE TANTRIC KISS

SOFT AND TENDER or full and passionate, the Tantric kiss is a profoundly intimate sexual exchange between two lovers. Kissing sensually awakens the erotic responses of the entire body and kindles the flame of passion. However, the Tantric kiss is not just a prelude to a bigger event, and it has no specific goal. Instead, it is valued for itself – a peak erotic experience of timelessness and merging. In Tantra, it is said that the exchange of body fluids through the saliva, which occurs in deep and intimate kissing, harmonizes and balances the male and female cosmic energies. Kissing deeply, the lovers' mouths symbolize the divine union of the Tantric deities, Shiva and Shakti, in blissful coitus: the soft yielding of the lips is like the softness of the female yoni, or vulva, and the penetrative action of the tongue corresponds to the penetration of the male lingam, or phallus.

"... he should *drink heavily* from her *lips* ..." THE KALACHAKRA TANTRA

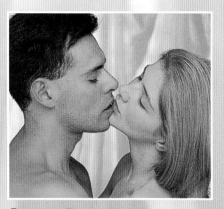 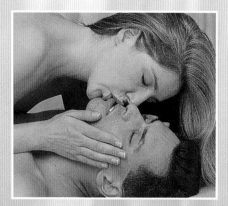 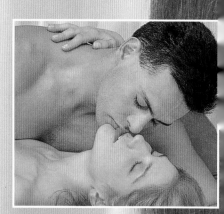

GENTLE EXPLORATION
Never rush into a full penetrative kiss. Let your mouths and tongues first gently play with each other. Place small tender kisses along your lover's upper and lower lips, and run the tip of your tongue sensuously over their moist softness. Through Tantric kissing, try to find a balanced exchange between your active and passive roles.

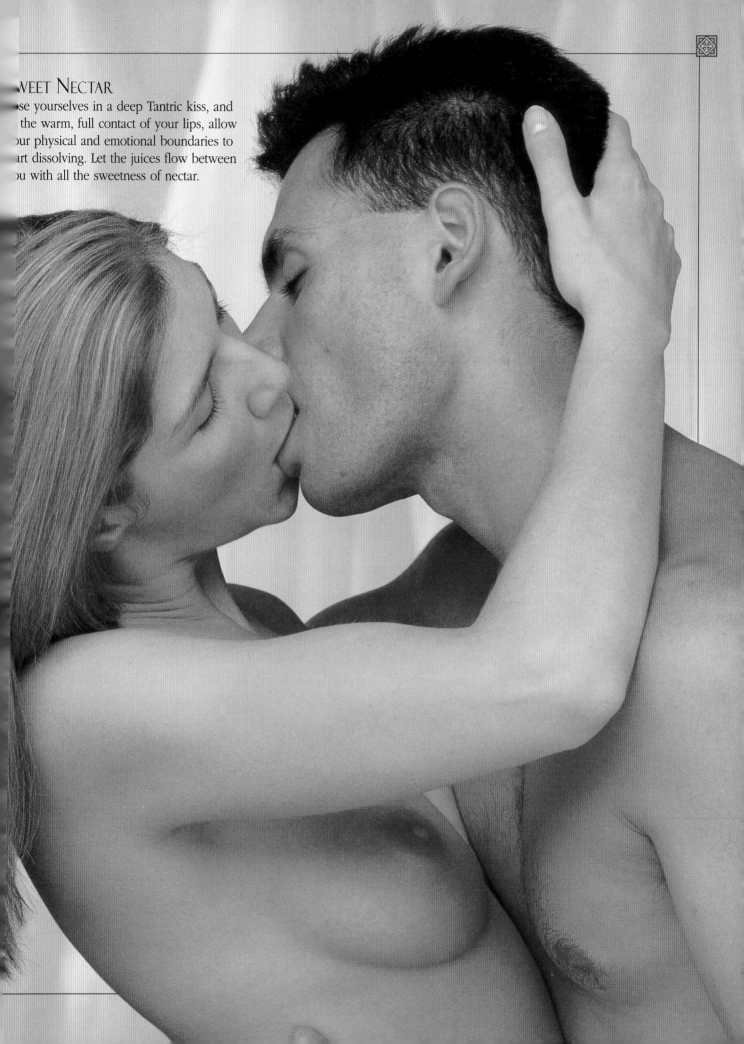

SWEET NECTAR

...se yourselves in a deep Tantric kiss, and ...the warm, full contact of your lips, allow ...ur physical and emotional boundaries to ...rt dissolving. Let the juices flow between ...ou with all the sweetness of nectar.

THE EROTIC BODY

DURING TRADITIONAL TANTRIC RITUALS, before a couple united in lovemaking, the male disciple performed an act of worship on his partner's body. Reciting a mantra of deep reverence, he touched each part of her body, starting from the right foot and moving up to her head, then descending to her left foot. In doing this, the man acknowledged the divinity residing within his woman, and saw in her the embodiment of the goddess Shakti. Imitate this ritual to honor your partner's entire body, cherishing every inch of skin with your hands, lips, and tongue. Never rush into intercourse, but slowly arouse the full eroticism of the body. By doing so, you will begin to harmonize not only your physical responses, but your hearts, minds, and feelings too.

"Her slower *excitement* demands *prolonged embraces* ..." ANANGA RANGA

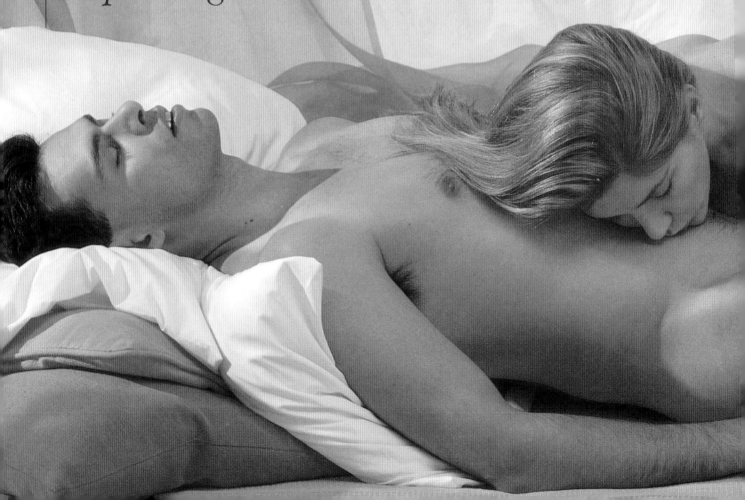

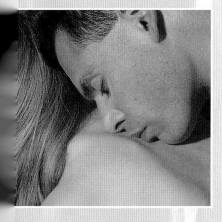
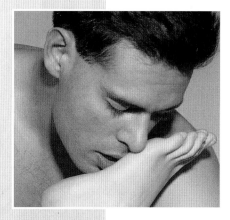
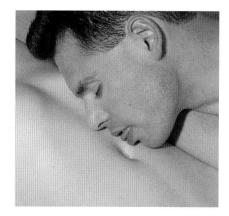
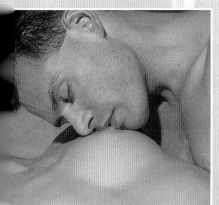
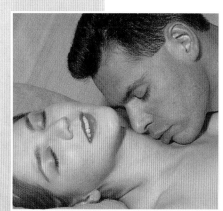
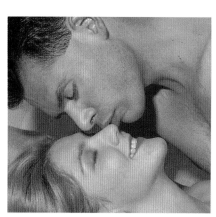
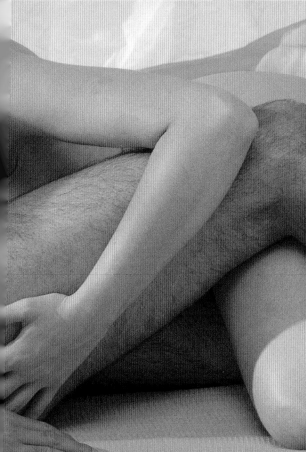

THE ALTAR OF LOVE △

A woman's whole body is responsive to sexual stimulation. According to ancient Tantric texts, the sensitivity of the female erogenous zones changes in relation to each phase of the lunar cycle. Remember, however, that each person is unique, and that only by enjoying touch and prolonged foreplay for its own sake can you discover your beloved's most erotic places and learn which caresses she finds most pleasing. Worship your woman from head to toe, taking the time to awaken the full eroticism of her body. Honor your lover's body as the Altar of Love.

◁ AWAKENING SENSUALITY

A man's most erogenous zone is his genital area. Stimulation in this region will rapidly arouse his profound sexual desire. However, your partner will also relish your kisses, caresses, and touches over his entire body, and they will enable him to channel his feelings into whole body sensuality.

BALANCING ENERGIES

A SUBTLE EXCHANGE of vital life force occurs between you and your beloved when you use your mouth and tongue to lovingly stimulate each other's sex organs. According to ancient Tantric texts, which detail the metaphysics of sexuality, mutual oral sex deepens the bond between lovers by balancing and harmonizing the polar masculine and feminine energies. Tantra calls the sexual secretions, "Love Juices," and regards them as a potent source of spiritual nourishment when they are absorbed orally in a respectful manner.

THE CROW

The oral sex position known as "69," called "The Crow" ancient Hindu scriptures, le the man and the woman enj fellatio and cunnilingus at the same time. A natural circuit psychic energy is created by the inverted position of both partners and by the intimate mouth to genital contact.

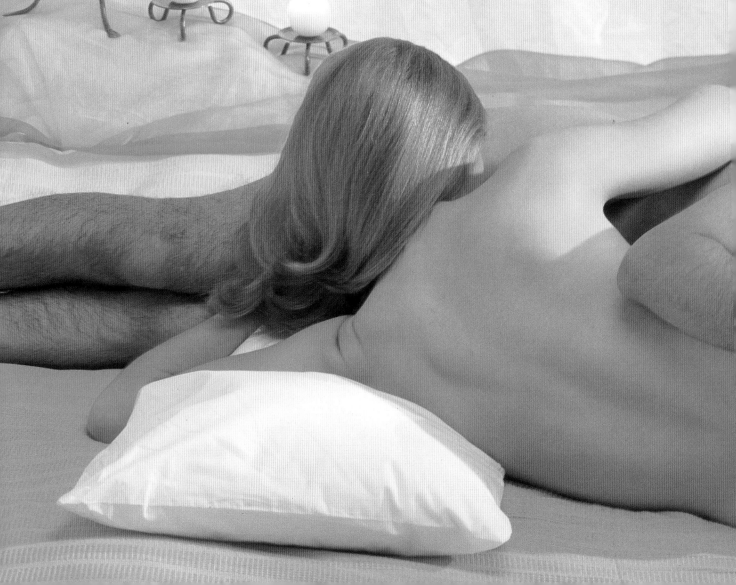

LOTUS NECTAR

In Tantra, a woman's vaginal secretions are considered to possess life-enhancing properties for the man when combined with saliva during oral sex. These juices are known as the Lotus Nectar. Kiss and lick her yoni with your lips and tongue to ecstatically arouse your beloved, and savor her sacred elixir as you do so.

REVERENCE

Take his penis into the luxurious softness of your mouth, flicking your tongue delicately along the length of its shaft and across its tip. Ask him to tell you which movements most arouse him. Tantra regards the emission of semen as wasteful unless the fellatio is practiced in an atmosphere of love, respect, and reverence.

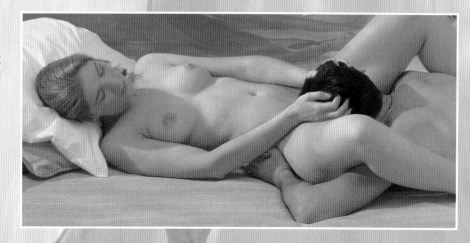

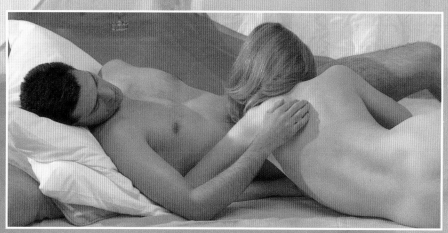

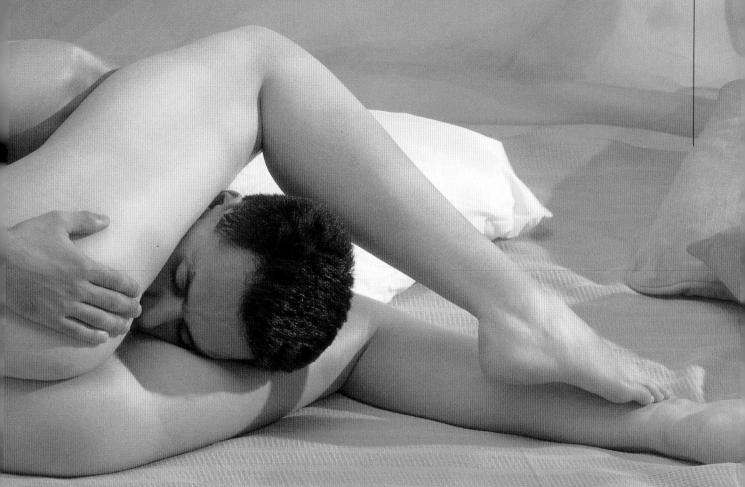

THE MASCULINE PRINCIPLE

WHEN THE MAN takes the dominant role in lovemaking, he is able to experience his strength and assertiveness in the sexual situation, and this can act as a powerful aphrodisiac for both sexes. However, at the same time, he should remain aware and sensitive to the needs of his partner and conscious of her pleasure. By allowing this combination of tenderness and power to occur, the man is realizing his "Shiva" potential: the active "solar" aspect of his masculinity that complements perfectly the passive "lunar" aspect of the woman's femininity.

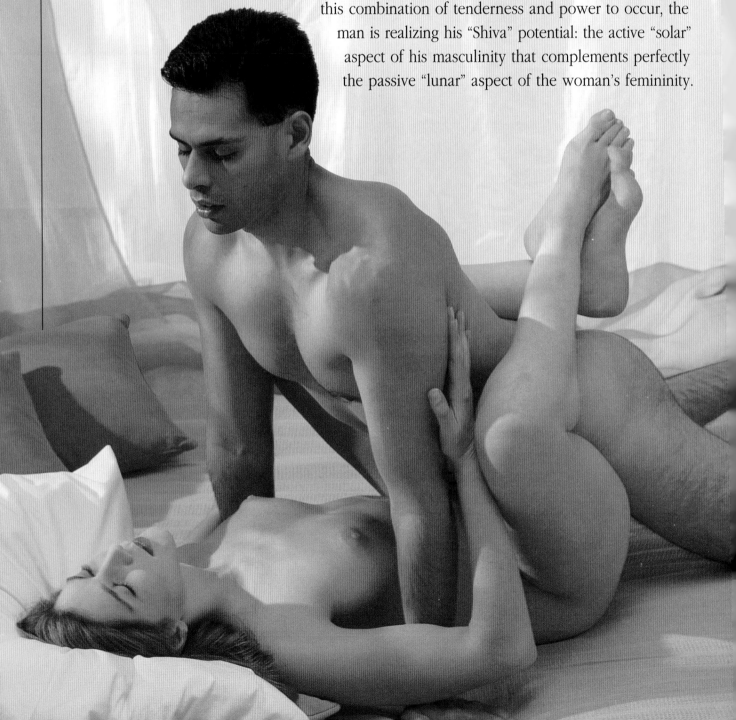

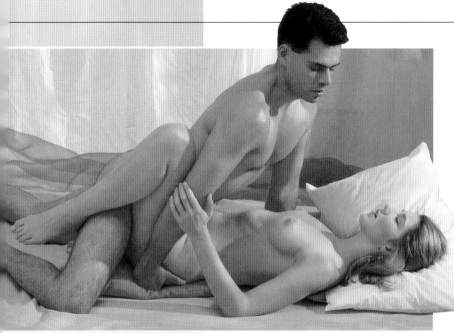

BE CONSIDERATE

Be aware of the woman's comfort at all times. Support your own weight and, when necessary, slip a pillow beneath her hips to ease the pressure on her pelvis. Penetrate your lover deeply only if she is fully aroused and her vagina is sufficiently lubricated to easily welcome and accommodate your penis. A wide variety of sexual movements and positions add to the interest and joy of your lovemaking (as long as you remain comfortable at all times). But be sure that your partner receives both vaginal and clitoral stimulation.

"*All the gods* worship that lingam, symbol of the Lord *Shiva*..." MAHABHARATA

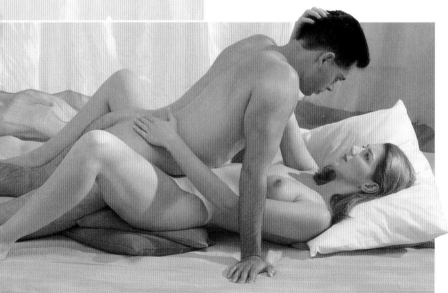

STAYING COOL

Try to avoid overexcitement, which propels you toward early orgasm, especially if your partner has not yet attained her own orgasm threshold. Take the pressure out of the situation by stopping or slowing activity well before you reach the "point of no return," withdrawing from your partner slightly so that only the tip of your penis remains inside her. Breathe slowly and deeply into your abdomen, and relax the muscles surrounding your genitals and anus.

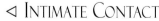

◁ INTIMATE CONTACT

The man-on-top "missionary" position is a very popular sexual position; it allows Tantric partners face-to-face and whole-body contact during lovemaking. The man has more freedom of movement and can easily vary the depth of penetration and the pace of thrusting. Likewise, the woman can use her legs to embrace her partner and draw him closer to her.

PLAYFUL DANCE

The more time you dedicate to making love with your partner, the more sexually compatible you will become. Familiarity with each other's body, rhythm, and pattern of response enhances the fluidity of your movements. As the man, you may like to take charge of initiating movement from one position to another. But take care that you do not turn this into a mechanical or gymnastic performance. Instead, try to remain spontaneous and playful at all times, so that the synchronicity of your lovemaking develops naturally and gracefully, like a beautiful dance.

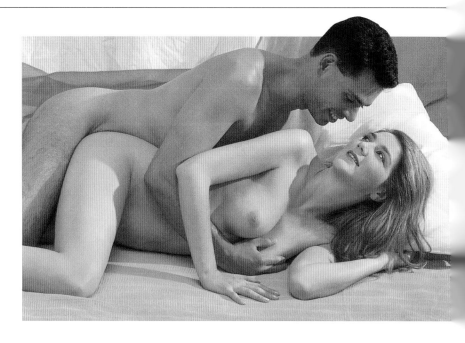

"Behold the Shiva Lingam...
firm as the Himalaya mountain,
tender as a folded leaf..." LINGA PURANA

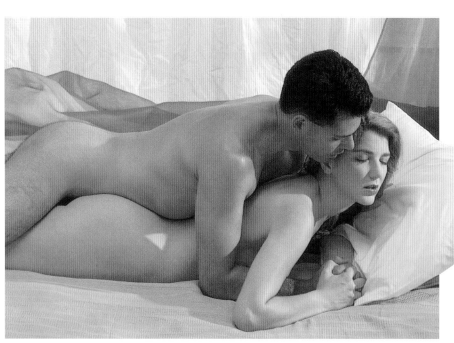

DOMINANT THEME

Certain sexual positions exaggerate the themes of domination and submission in lovemaking. The adoption of erotic postures can be equally pleasurable to the man and woman. The Tantric sexual position that is shown here, known as the Elephant posture, is described in several ancient Hindu texts. While supporting his own weight, the man lies over the length of the woman's body and enters her vagina from the rear. The woman is then able to tighten her thighs and wriggle her hips to greatly enhance their mutual arousal.

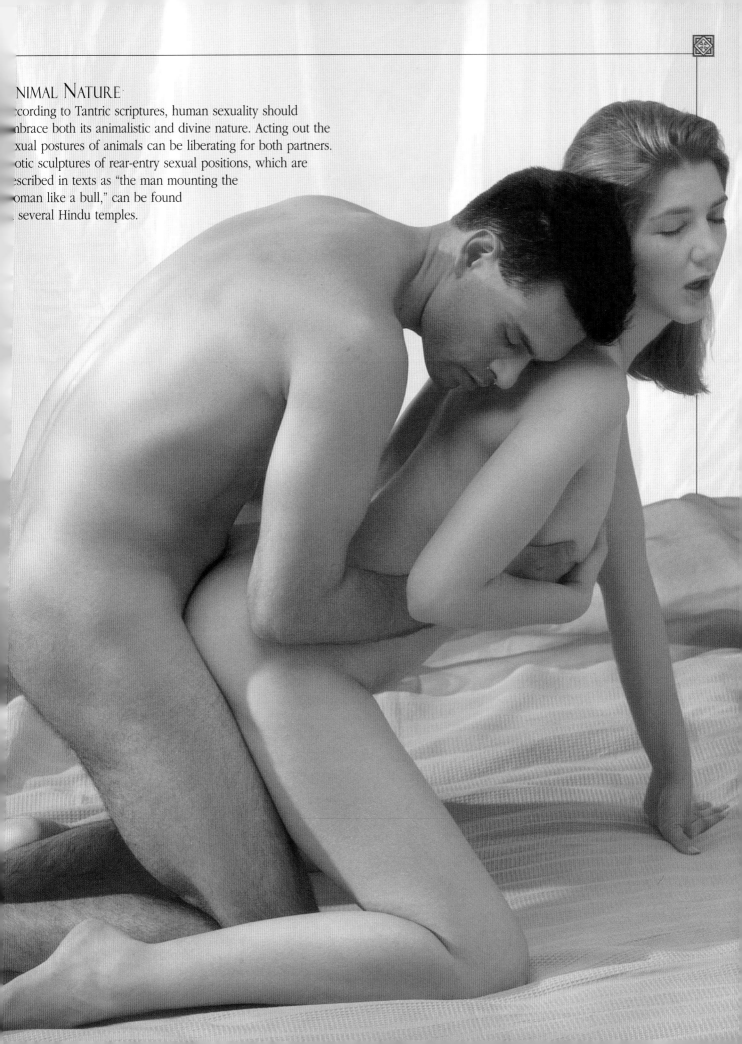

ANIMAL NATURE

According to Tantric scriptures, human sexuality should embrace both its animalistic and divine nature. Acting out the sexual postures of animals can be liberating for both partners. Erotic sculptures of rear-entry sexual positions, which are described in texts as "the man mounting the woman like a bull," can be found in several Hindu temples.

CAPTURING THE MOMENT

HOWEVER PASSIONATE your sexual activity is, slow down occasionally and simply *be* with each other. When you feel you are emotionally losing contact with your partner, whether because you are lost in your own thoughts and fantasies or are too busy with activity and technique, then consciously bring yourself back into the moment and reconnect with your beloved. By allowing stillness and non-doing to be part of your sexual union, you can capture those moments through which you are able to glimpse the very essence of Tantra. B letting your tender feelings come to the surface, you reveal your vulnerability and sweetness to each other. Slowing down enables you to recuperate your energies, and to savor your precious time together instead of rushing toward a speedy climax.

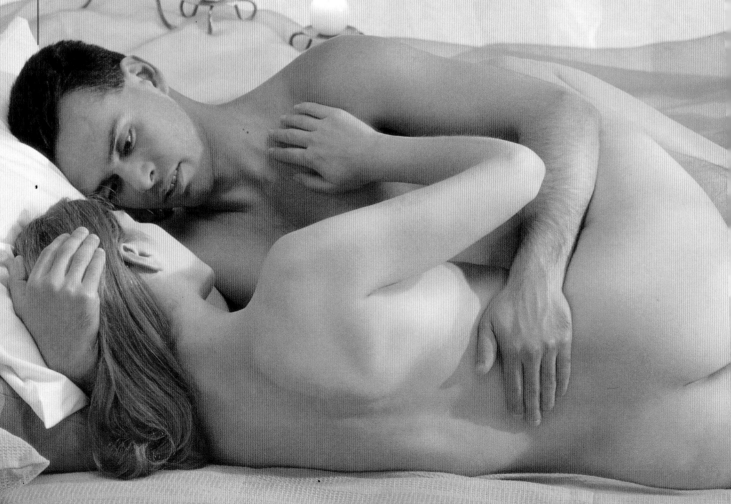

KEEPING CONTACT

When slowing down during passionate lovemaking, keep the intimacy of your contact alive by looking into each other's eyes. Gaze at one another with love, seeing deep within your lover's soul. Fall into the moment, harmonizing your breathing and becoming aware of the closeness and warmth of your bodies.

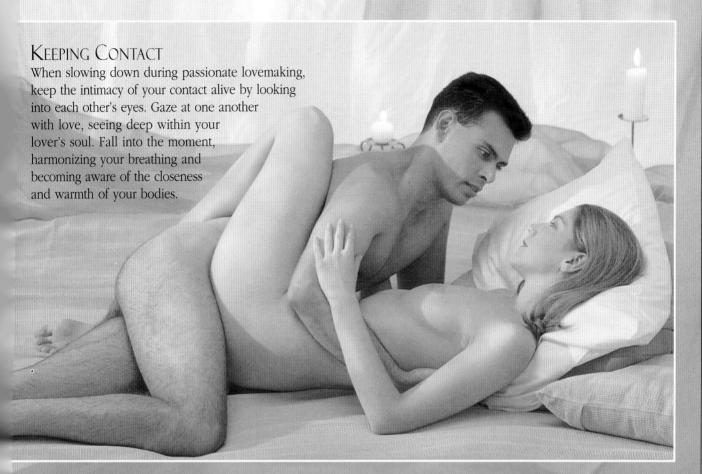

"The *Goddess* resides in *all women* and the *Lord* abides in *all men*." JVALAVALI VAJRAMALA

STILL TOGETHER

Rolling over into this side-by-side position enables you to rest while remaining in coitus. Look at each other and breathe together, and whenever the male partner needs stimulation to maintain his erection, the woman can gently undulate her hips. Allow the next wave of sexual intensity to arise spontaneously.

THE FEMININE PRINCIPLE

A WOMAN'S SEXUAL HAPPINESS and fulfillment is of paramount importance to Tantric lovemaking. She is equal in all things, and, indeed, the woman is regarded as the initiator and kinetic force of the sexual energy. According to Tantra, no man can be sexually satisfied unless his woman is filled with joy from the union. It is important to experiment with exchanging roles while making love, giving the female partner the freedom to express herself sexually both in the active and passive positions. Switching roles also allows the man to experience the beauty of surrendering himself to her erotic feminine power.

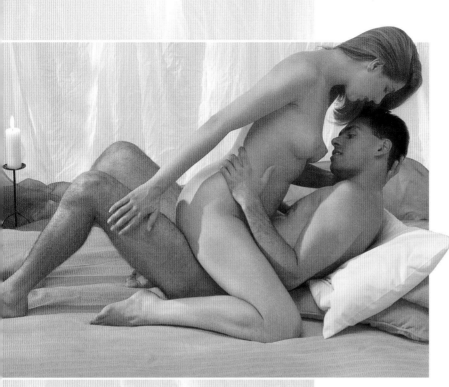

SWEET OFFERING

When you have taken the active, on-top position, you are able to reveal the full and sensual form of your body to your partner, offering to him your breast so that he can tenderly kiss and suck it. This gesture will be very pleasing to him, and as his lips and tongue caress your nipple, it will also heighten your own state of arousal. The breasts are highly erogenous, and sensual stimulation of them will activate the emotional and sexual centers in your brain. By offering your breasts, you symbolize the essence of womanhood, embodying the universal lover and mother in one.

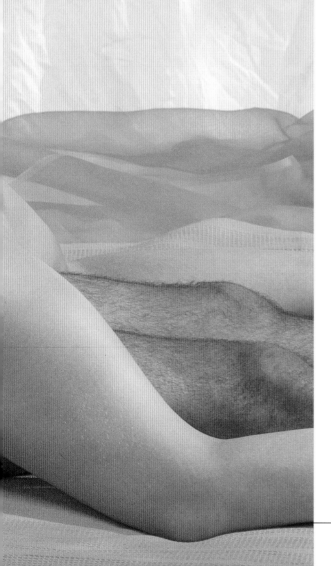

"A woman is the *supreme initiatress* of Tantra." KAULARAHASYA

INITIATING PLEASURE

In the active sexual role, you can enjoy freedom of movement as well as control over the pace, rhythm, and depth of penetrative sex. You can also position yourself so as to receive maximum arousal by bringing your vulva close to his pubic bone. Harmonize your own joy with your lover's pleasure by staying sensitive and in tune with his responses. Taking the on-top position can help your male partner to become more relaxed and thus prolong the lovemaking phase before he ejaculates.

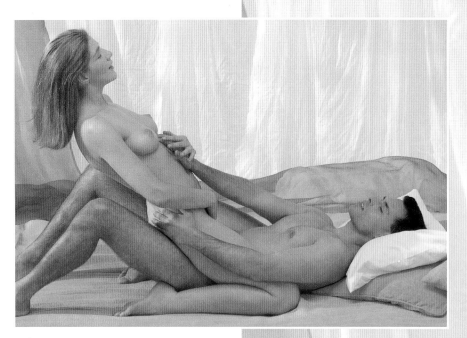

◁ EROTIC PLACES

Increase your own erotic arousal by sensually touching your clitoris while, at the same time, bringing happiness your partner. Lean back and move yo pelvis so his penis presses and rubs against the front wall of your vagina. Located here is the G-spot, a small, highly erotogenic area situated about three finger widths above the pubic bone. For many women, pressure on this zone intensifies orgasm.

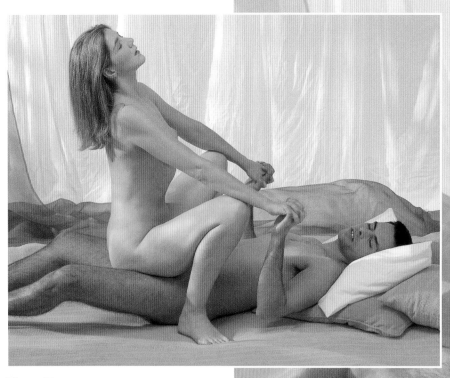

KALI POSTURE △

This squatting position replicates the Tantric image of the goddess Kali seated in intercourse on the body of her inert husband, Shiva. It gives you the freedom to rotate your pelvis while his penis penetrates you deeply. Lower yourself carefully onto his penis to avoid hurting your partner.

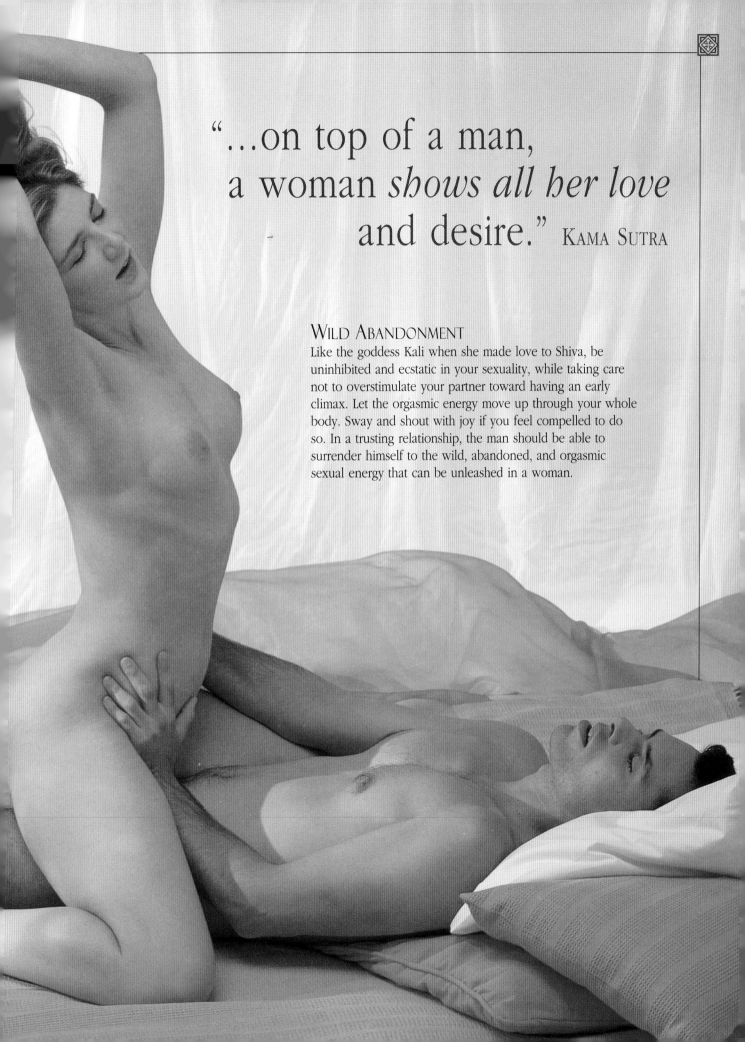

"...on top of a man, a woman *shows all her love and desire.*" KAMA SUTRA

WILD ABANDONMENT

Like the goddess Kali when she made love to Shiva, be uninhibited and ecstatic in your sexuality, while taking care not to overstimulate your partner toward having an early climax. Let the orgasmic energy move up through your whole body. Sway and shout with joy if you feel compelled to do so. In a trusting relationship, the man should be able to surrender himself to the wild, abandoned, and orgasmic sexual energy that can be unleashed in a woman.

THE ORGASMIC WAVE

TANTRIC LOVERS do not pursue orgasm as the only goal of lovemaking but, instead, use the orgasmic energy as a force for transforming their sexual relationship. The less effort involved, the more fulfilling your experience will be. Stay in the moment when making love, and submerge yourselves totally into each sensual experience. As the orgasmic tension increases, relax and breathe together, allowing the waves of pleasure to build up and permeate your whole body. Avoid rushing headlong to the point of no return, but savor the plateau phase that precedes the climax. By consciously riding the crest of the wave, the man can endeavor to wait for the woman to reach her orgasmic peak.

SURRENDER TO JOY
When the orgasmic waves have reached their crescendo for both of you, you can then relinquish all control over your breath, body, and mind. Allow the waves to surge through your bodies from head to toe and surrender yourselves completely to their powerful pulsations. Let go of inhibition and express your joy.

"The *sexual* activity of Shiva and Shakti makes the *moon wax* and *wane*." SHIVA PURANA

THE ORGASMIC CYCLE
Learn to understand and respond to each other's physical and emotional needs while making love. By harmonizing the basic sexual differences that occur in your patterns of arousal and orgasm, you can achieve a more compatible level of sexual happiness. There are four phases to the orgasmic cycle for both sexes: arousal, plateau, climax, and resolution. However, men and women do differ in their responses during each phase. Men are more likely to be aroused faster than women, have a shorter plateau phase before orgasm, and need a longer resolution period after climaxing. To attain greater orgasmic satisfaction, take the time to discuss your sexual differences and commit quality time to foreplay and lovemaking for its own sake.

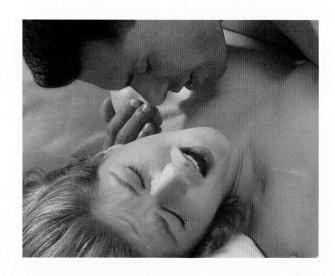

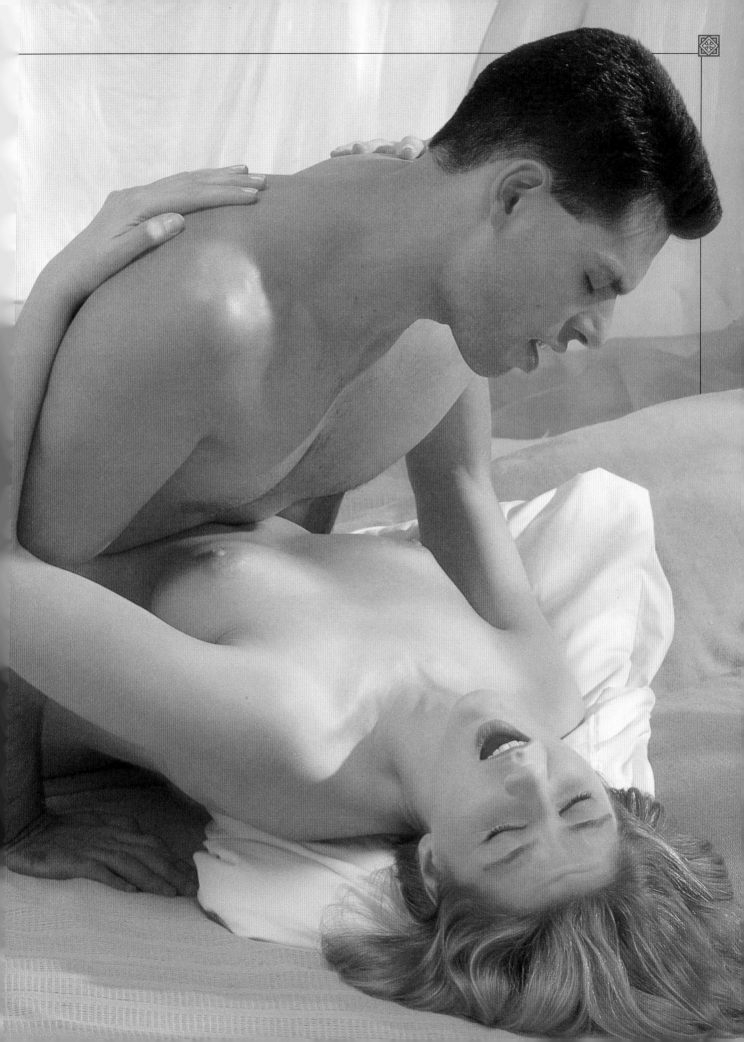

STAYING CONNECTED

THE MOMENTS that follow sexual activity can be very precious if both partners are able to treasure the stillness and sense of merging that becomes manifest in the wake of orgasm or the completion of sexual intercourse. According to Tantric teaching, it is then that your energies can fuse and find a state of equilibrium, so that later you feel refreshed and replenished by your sexual communion. Do not rush away from your sacred lovemaking space, but relax totally and lie in each other's arms. Never shower immediately after intercourse, but let your love juices mingle together.

A VULNERABLE TIME

When a man has ejaculated his semen, he may feel tired and depleted for a while. Conversely, the woman may feel energized and want more tactile contact. This can cause a misunderstanding between you at the very time when you should be at your most intimate and vulnerable with each other. Rather than cutting off, or becoming frustrated, seek to understand and accommodate your different needs during this sensitive resolution period.

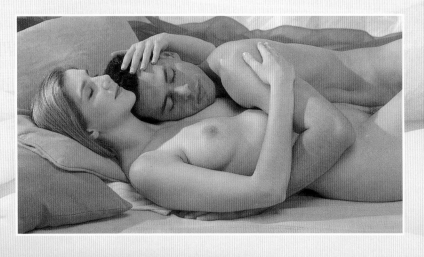

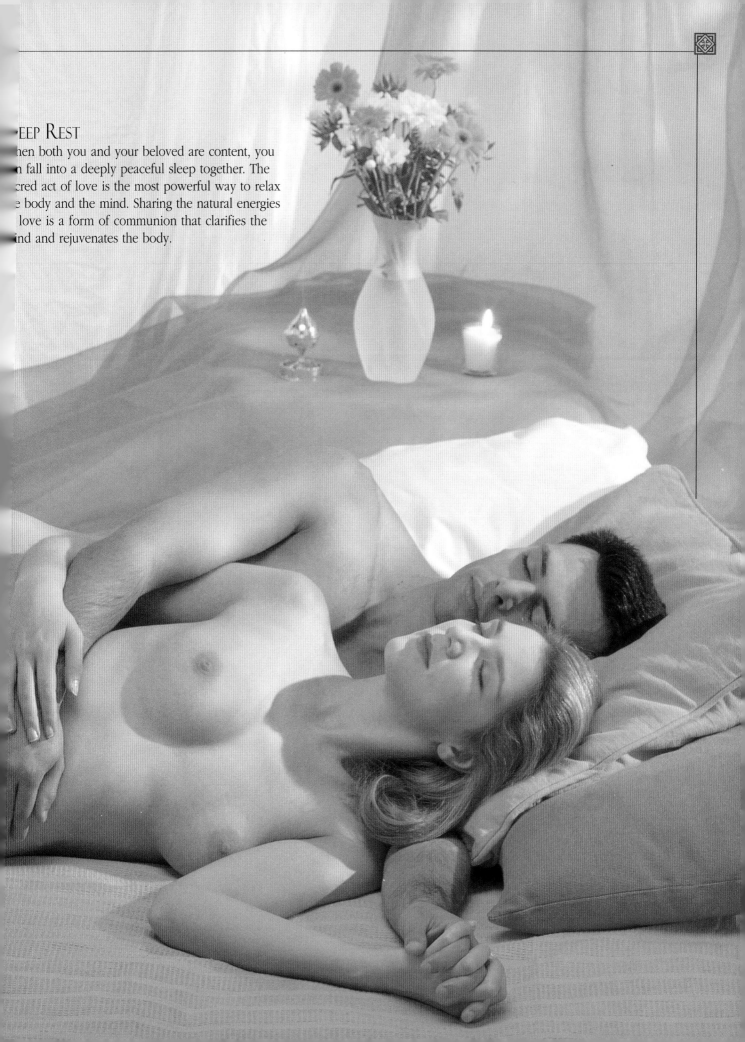

EEP REST

hen both you and your beloved are content, you
n fall into a deeply peaceful sleep together. The
cred act of love is the most powerful way to relax
e body and the mind. Sharing the natural energies
love is a form of communion that clarifies the
ind and rejuvenates the body.

STRENGTHENING THE TEMPLE OF THE SPIRIT

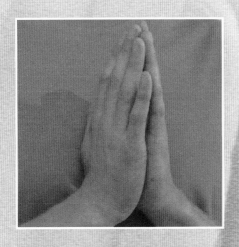

"*There is but one temple in the universe, and that is the body of man. Nothing is holier than that high form*"

NOVALIS

THE TEMPLES OF INDIA WERE TRADITIONALLY BUILT TO SYMBOLICALLY REPRESENT THE STRUCTURE OF

the human body. Different areas of the temple were given the

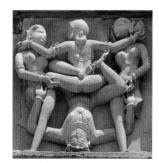

names of human body parts. For example, the top of the temple is the head, and the INNER *sanctuary* is the womb.

Complex sexo-yogic postures adorn the walls of temples in Khajuraho, India.

Conversely, the sages of India referred to the human body as the Temple of the Spirit. The reverence accorded to the body is encapsulated in the words of the mystic Saraha Doha: "I have not encountered another TEMPLE *that is as blissful* as my own body." Gaining respect for your body and strengthening it through routine stretch exercises, or Hatha Yoga postures known as asanas, will become a valuable part of your Tantric practice.

THIS CHAPTER introduces you to some basic yoga asanas, stretch and movement exercises designed to bring STABILITY *and suppleness* to your body, particularly to those areas that affect sexual vitality. If you wish to gain a greater understanding of the science of Hatha Yoga, you should study the postures from a book dedicated to the subject, under the guidance of a qualified Hatha Yoga teacher. Do not attempt advanced yogic asanas without expert tuition.

TANTRIC TEXTS have always embraced the ancient sciences of both Hatha Yoga and Kundalini Yoga, not only as a physical aid to attaining complex Tantric sexual postures but also as a means of UNIFYING *body and spirit* and of harmonizing and channeling Kundalini energy. It is crucial to have physical stability and fluidity of motion to allow sexual energy to move spontaneously and joyfully through your body, and between you and your lover.

Always stretch and warm your muscles before beginning an exercise program.

ENDEAVOR, TOGETHER with your Tantric partner, to commit yourself to a regular stretch and yoga program, combined with pranayama exercises and meditation (*see p.102*). Enter your sacred space to practice your yogic asanas at SUNRISE *or sunset,* if possible. Wear loose-fitting cotton clothing, and use special yoga exercise mats. Have some cushions close by for added comfort and support. Remember that it is far better to do a little exercise every day rather than a marathon session once a week. In a matter of weeks you will feel the enormous benefits of the time and effort you invest.

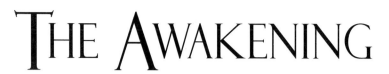

THE AWAKENING

AWAKEN EARLY with your partner to welcome the rising sun and absorb its life-giving properties. Perform two rounds of the Sun Salutation – a 12-step cycle of yoga stretches, which balances body and mind through the integration of movement and breath. Inhale on each extension, and exhale on each contraction. Learn the full set of movements with a yoga teacher to move gracefully and without strain.

12 Exhale slowly, droppi... your arms down to your s... while maintaining a sense... lift throughout your entire... You are now ... to repeat the c...

11 On the inhalation, lift your arms into the air, and stand with a straight back. Relax your shoulders and neck.

10 This step is a repeat of stage 3. Exhale and bring your left foot back up to meet the front foot, straighten your legs as much as possible, and tuck your chin into your chest.

9 Inhale and bring your right knee into the chest while keeping the left leg and the arms straight. Keep your head raised and your spine flat.

8 Exhale steadily. Keep your spine straight and support your weight on your hands and toes. Straighten your arms to raise yourself up into the familiar "push-up" position.

7 Exhale as you drop your head to straighten the spine, then inhale and tuck your toes under your body as you prepare to raise yourself up.

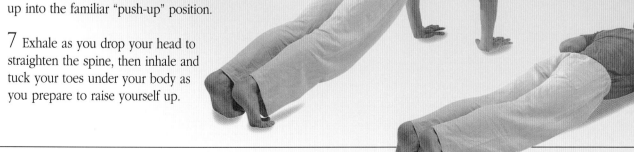

Stand with your feet together and take a deep breath. Exhale slowly as you bring your hands together at the chest into the prayer position.

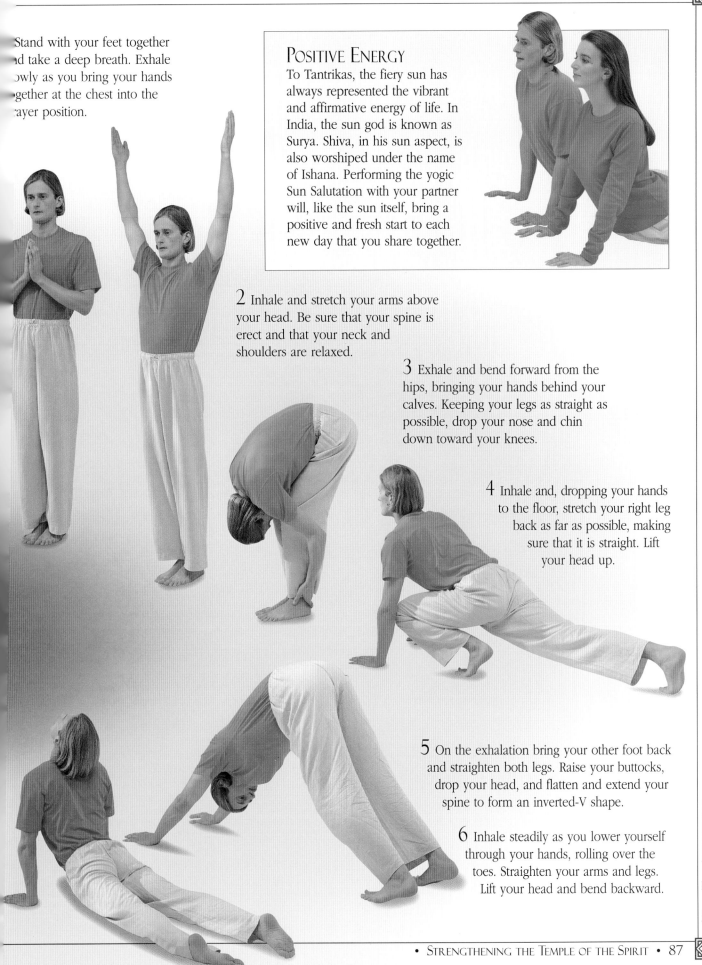

POSITIVE ENERGY

To Tantrikas, the fiery sun has always represented the vibrant and affirmative energy of life. In India, the sun god is known as Surya. Shiva, in his sun aspect, is also worshiped under the name of Ishana. Performing the yogic Sun Salutation with your partner will, like the sun itself, bring a positive and fresh start to each new day that you share together.

2 Inhale and stretch your arms above your head. Be sure that your spine is erect and that your neck and shoulders are relaxed.

3 Exhale and bend forward from the hips, bringing your hands behind your calves. Keeping your legs as straight as possible, drop your nose and chin down toward your knees.

4 Inhale and, dropping your hands to the floor, stretch your right leg back as far as possible, making sure that it is straight. Lift your head up.

5 On the exhalation bring your other foot back and straighten both legs. Raise your buttocks, drop your head, and flatten and extend your spine to form an inverted-V shape.

6 Inhale steadily as you lower yourself through your hands, rolling over the toes. Straighten your arms and legs. Lift your head and bend backward.

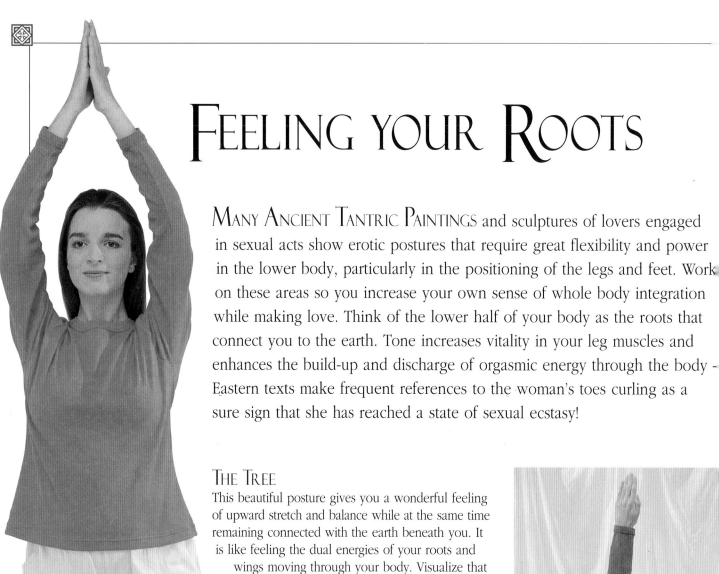

FEELING YOUR ROOTS

MANY ANCIENT TANTRIC PAINTINGS and sculptures of lovers engaged in sexual acts show erotic postures that require great flexibility and power in the lower body, particularly in the positioning of the legs and feet. Work on these areas so you increase your own sense of whole body integration while making love. Think of the lower half of your body as the roots that connect you to the earth. Tone increases vitality in your leg muscles and enhances the build-up and discharge of orgasmic energy through the body - Eastern texts make frequent references to the woman's toes curling as a sure sign that she has reached a state of sexual ecstasy!

THE TREE
This beautiful posture gives you a wonderful feeling of upward stretch and balance while at the same time remaining connected with the earth beneath you. It is like feeling the dual energies of your roots and wings moving through your body. Visualize that your heel is actually extending down into the earth like a root. It will help you to remain stable and firm on the supporting leg. Press the sole of the other foot flat against the top of the inner thigh, keeping the knee aligned to your hips. Breathe deeply and repeat on the other side.

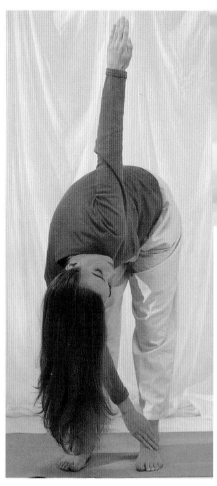

TOE TOUCHING ▷
Adopt this posture to relax your body and refresh your mind. Take a deep breath and, on the outward breath, bend forward slowly from the hip, keeping the back and legs as straight as possible. Be sure the body relaxes while you work the legs. Feel the stretch through your legs, particularly on the backs of your thighs and in your calf muscles. Hold for five seconds, then repeat the exercise on the other side.

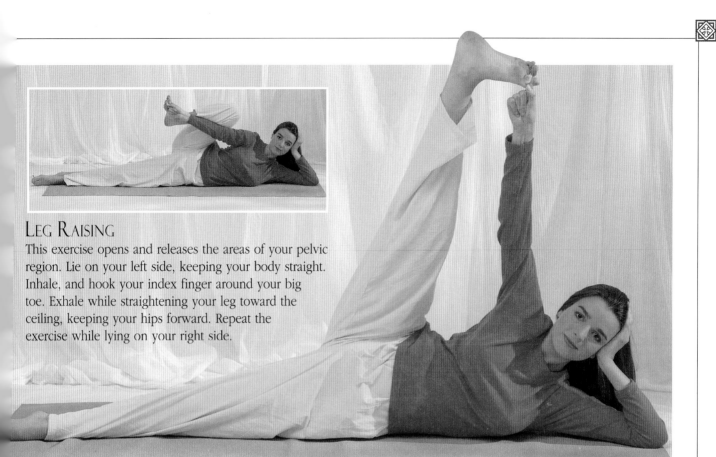

LEG RAISING

This exercise opens and releases the areas of your pelvic region. Lie on your left side, keeping your body straight. Inhale, and hook your index finger around your big toe. Exhale while straightening your leg toward the ceiling, keeping your hips forward. Repeat the exercise while lying on your right side.

"*Calmness and steadiness* of the body are known as Yoga." KATHA UPANISHAD

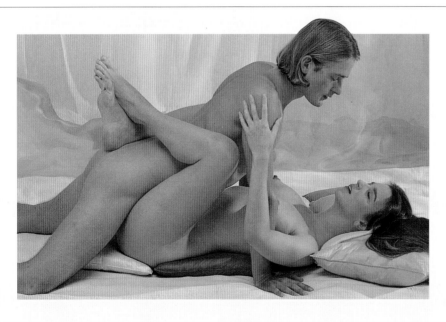

FEELING STRONG

Strong but flexible leg muscles increase your feeling of power during lovemaking and enhance your control over lovemaking positions. When the woman is lying on her back she can use her legs to hold the man or pull him toward her, crossing her legs easily behind his back for more intimate contact. Strength in the man's legs enables him to move more easily while supporting his own weight and, in some postures, the weight of his lover.

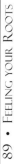

FREEING THE SEXUAL WAVE

ORGASMIC ENERGY moves like a wave through the body unless it is impeded by physical or emotional tensions. By relaxing tight contracted muscles through stretch and yoga postures, you can free areas, such as the pelvis and spine, which are vital to the expression of your sexuality. The Sushumna, which is the channel in the subtle body through which the Kundalini energy ascends, is represented in the physical body by the spinal column. These exercises help keep your spine flexible – a healthy spine is as vital to your spiritual and sexual well-being as it is to your physical well-being.

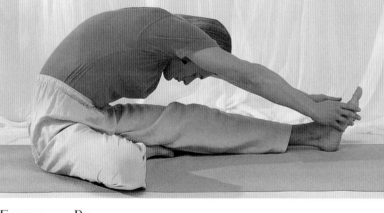

FORWARD BEND
This body stretch soothes the mind while working the spinal column, heart, and abdomen. Raise your arms as you extend your torso upward. On an exhalation, gently extend your chest toward your knees as you reach for your foot. Hold for a few seconds and then relax. Repeat on the other side.

SPINAL TWIST
The upper body twist energizes you by freeing tension in the spine. With your knees forward and spine extended, take your right arm across your left thigh and place your left arm behind your back. Breathe deeply and, on an exhalation, twist gently to the right. Release, and repeat on the other side.

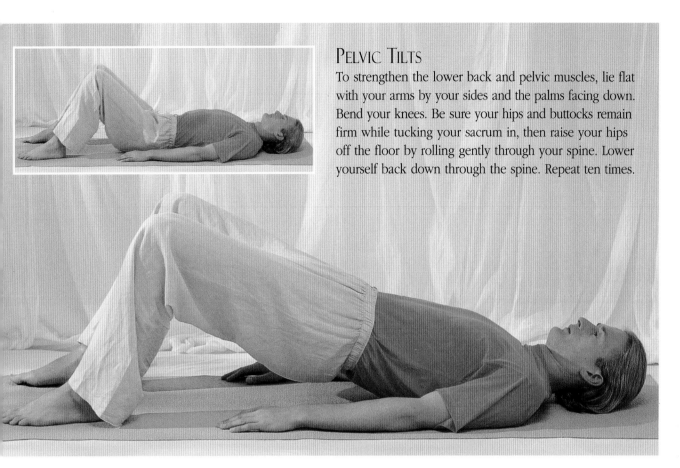

PELVIC TILTS

To strengthen the lower back and pelvic muscles, lie flat with your arms by your sides and the palms facing down. Bend your knees. Be sure your hips and buttocks remain firm while tucking your sacrum in, then raise your hips off the floor by rolling gently through your spine. Lower yourself back down through the spine. Repeat ten times.

"Bliss is *ever-rising* due to the union of Shiva and Shakti." SHIVA PURANA

PULSATING ENERGY

Lovemaking movements become graceful and refined when there is flexibility in the pelvis and spine. The woman can enjoy sensually rotating her pelvis in the on-top position, and her partner can respond with subtle thrusting motions. Orgasmic sensations can flow more freely and pulsate through the whole body, enabling lovers to surrender to each other body, heart, and soul.

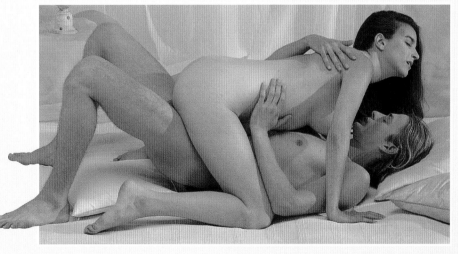

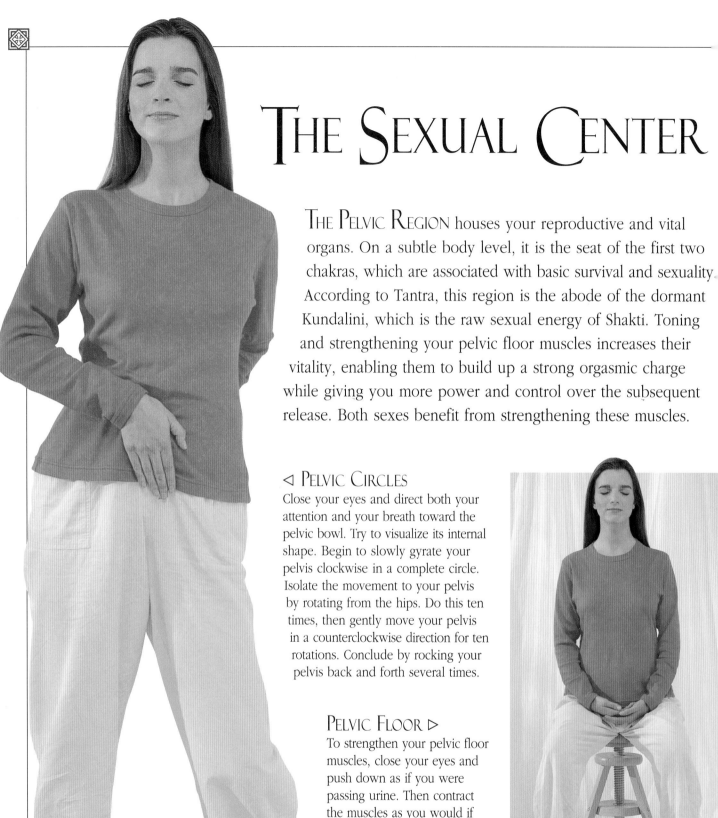

THE SEXUAL CENTER

THE PELVIC REGION houses your reproductive and vital organs. On a subtle body level, it is the seat of the first two chakras, which are associated with basic survival and sexuality. According to Tantra, this region is the abode of the dormant Kundalini, which is the raw sexual energy of Shakti. Toning and strengthening your pelvic floor muscles increases their vitality, enabling them to build up a strong orgasmic charge while giving you more power and control over the subsequent release. Both sexes benefit from strengthening these muscles.

◁ PELVIC CIRCLES
Close your eyes and direct both your attention and your breath toward the pelvic bowl. Try to visualize its internal shape. Begin to slowly gyrate your pelvis clockwise in a complete circle. Isolate the movement to your pelvis by rotating from the hips. Do this ten times, then gently move your pelvis in a counterclockwise direction for ten rotations. Conclude by rocking your pelvis back and forth several times.

PELVIC FLOOR ▷
To strengthen your pelvic floor muscles, close your eyes and push down as if you were passing urine. Then contract the muscles as you would if you were to stop the flow. Hold for a count of three, then release the muscles and repeat the process. This exercise can be performed either sitting or standing. Do ten repetitions, at least three times a day.

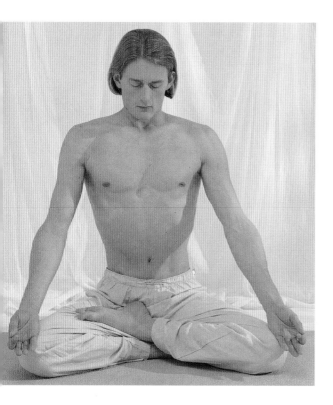

Mula Bandha - Anal Sphincter Control

Anal sphincter control is an advanced yogic technique used by Tantrikas to regulate the flow of semen. Lower your head and focus your attention into the pelvic region. Inhale, and consciously constrict the muscles around the anus for three sets of ten repetitions. The perineum, between the scrotum and anus, is the location of a duct through which ejaculated semen must pass. Perfection of the Mula Bandha effectively blocks this passage, so retaining semen during lovemaking.

"By *inner firmness* I have caused my *seed* to remain in my lingam…" SKANDA PURANA

Gaining Control

The woman can use her pelvic floor muscles to great erotic effect. By contracting and relaxing her vaginal walls to embrace and milk her partner's penis, she will greatly increase their mutual sexual delight. Likewise, she can also raise herself upward but still tantalizingly clasp the head of his penis. When the man has control over his pelvic muscles, through breathing and locking techniques such as the Mula Bandha (*see above*), he can draw sexual energy up and away from his genital area, so prolonging his lovemaking and intensifying the power of his ultimate orgasmic release.

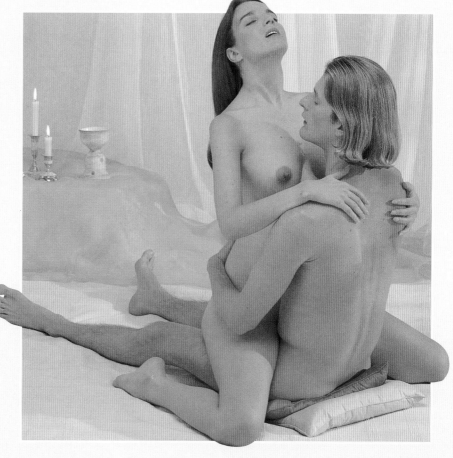

OPENING THE LOTUS

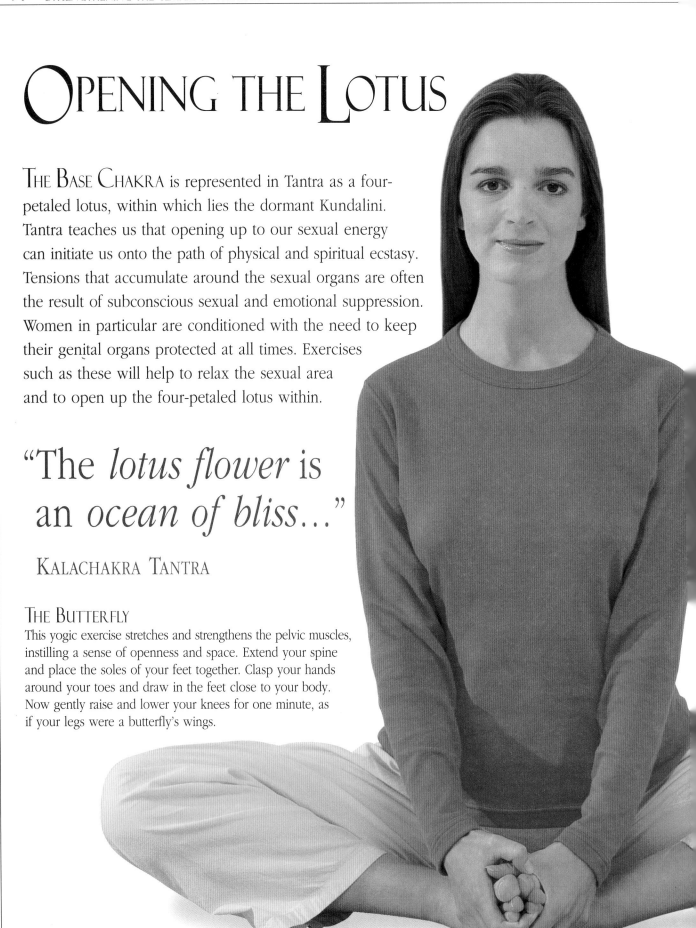

THE BASE CHAKRA is represented in Tantra as a four-petaled lotus, within which lies the dormant Kundalini. Tantra teaches us that opening up to our sexual energy can initiate us onto the path of physical and spiritual ecstasy. Tensions that accumulate around the sexual organs are often the result of subconscious sexual and emotional suppression. Women in particular are conditioned with the need to keep their genital organs protected at all times. Exercises such as these will help to relax the sexual area and to open up the four-petaled lotus within.

"The *lotus flower* is an *ocean of bliss...*"

KALACHAKRA TANTRA

THE BUTTERFLY

This yogic exercise stretches and strengthens the pelvic muscles, instilling a sense of openness and space. Extend your spine and place the soles of your feet together. Clasp your hands around your toes and draw in the feet close to your body. Now gently raise and lower your knees for one minute, as if your legs were a butterfly's wings.

YAWNING WIDE

This stretch removes fatigue and tension in the legs and opens the pelvic and groin region. Lying with your back flat against the floor and with your buttocks pressed against a wall, extend your legs up the wall. Allow the legs to spread gently apart. Relax and breathe deeply, holding the position for about one minute.

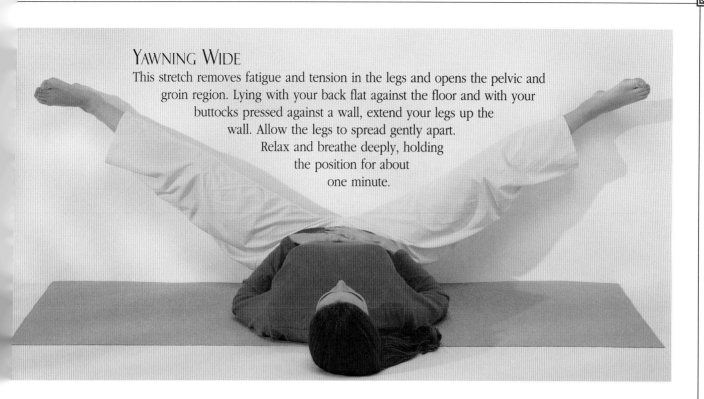

SEXUAL OPENNESS

It is a great joy to be sexually uninhibited, and to be able to surrender yourself to spontaneous erotic pleasure. When you feel sexually open, you are willing to experiment with your lovemaking. Here, the woman places a leg on each of her partner's shoulders and relaxes her pelvic muscles so he can penetrate her deeply. In the Chandamaharosana Tantra, an ancient Tantric text, this is known as the Mounted Yantra position.

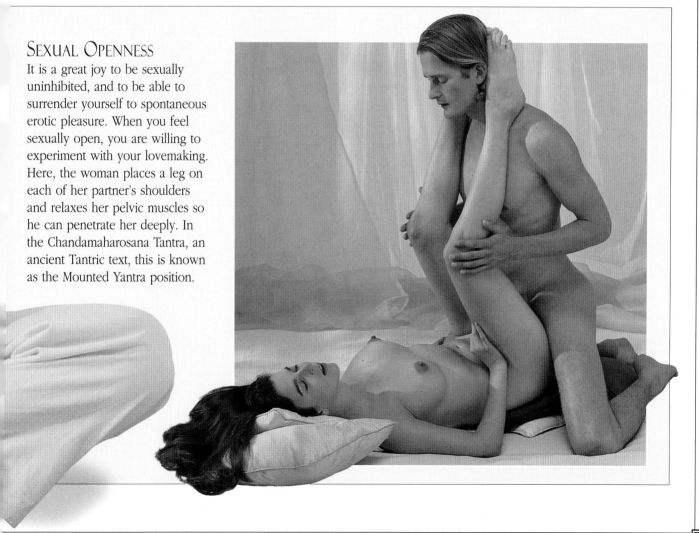

PURIFYING THE MIND, BODY & SPIRIT

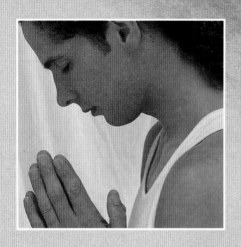

"With palms joined in reverence, the meditator shall retain the breath and sit down, with his mind and sense organs under full control. He shall then meditate on the chakras"

SHIVA PURANA

TANTRA ENCOURAGES YOU TO CELEBRATE LIFE TO THE FULL AND TO ENJOY SENSUAL PLEASURES

without inhibition. However, far from presenting a license for debauchery, as some Victorian interpreters of Tantric scriptures concluded, it is a discipline which demands that you develop a high degree of awareness and full PURITY *of intention.* It involves the transformation of body, mind, and spirit, stating that health and joy are achieved only when you are in HARMONY *within* yourself and in relation to the external world. A Tantric sexual relationship exists only when partners acquire a meditative quality of awareness.

Shiva and Parvati spent many years in the practice of meditation.

IN TRADITIONAL Tantra, disciples practiced meditation and pranayama for years, under the guidance of a spiritual teacher. In searching for SPIRITUAL *enlightenment,* they learned the sexo-yogic asanas necessary to focus the mind and steady the physical processes of the body. This chapter demonstrates how you, as a modern couple, can adapt these practices to achieve greater equilibrium in your BODY, *mind, and spirit.* It encourages you to incorporate pranayama and meditation practices as a natural part of your Tantric relationship.

BY PARTICIPATING in visualization exercises, energy work, chakra meditations, and Tantric massage, you will become more aware of the etheric body. This will increase your sensitivity toward yourself and your lover, and you will soon feel energy as a TANGIBLE *force* resonating within and around the body. As you become increasingly fine-tuned to this level of vibration, your lovemaking will be NATURALLY *transformed* into something more subtle, meditative, and Tantric.

Energy work will increase your responsiveness to your Tantric lover.

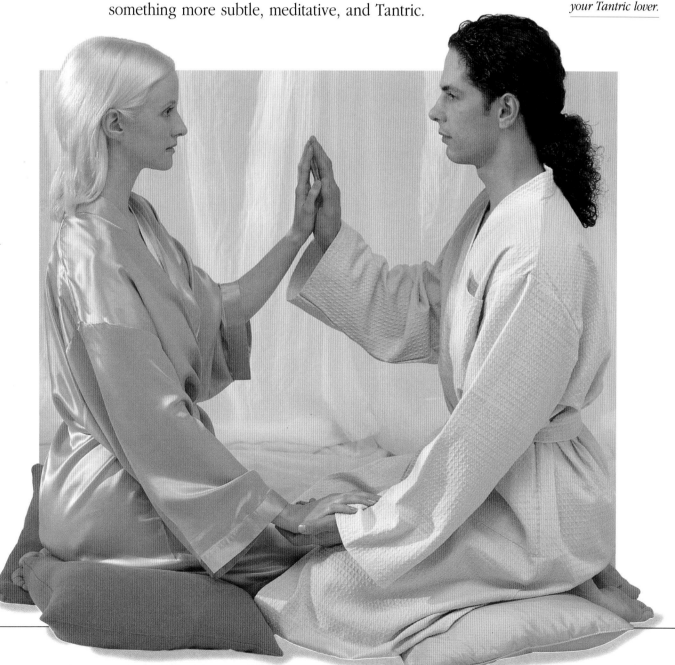

LIVING IN BALANCE

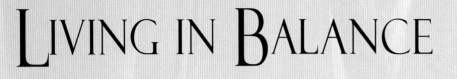

A TANTRIC LIFESTYLE celebrates the joys of life, but seeks to maintain a state of harmony within it. Health and happiness flourish when you bring greater awareness to all your daily activities. Find the right balance between rest and activity, pleasure and work, body and mind, intellect and spirit. Fundamental to this holistic approach is the food you eat. Food not only forms your physical body, but also influences your mind, thoughts, and emotions. It affects your sexual sensitivity, and even the taste and odor of sexual secretions. Yogic teaching divides food into three types: sattvic, rajasic, and tamasic. Understanding these categories can help you select foods that are purifying and enjoyable.

THREE QUALITIES

Sattvic foods are pure, inducing calm and meditative feelings. They include milk, honey, whole grains, fruits, nuts, nonroot vegetables, and legumes. Rajasic foods produce heat, inducing passion and mental overactivity. This category includes all spicy ingredients, such as onions and chili, and stimulants like tea and coffee. Chicken, fish, and root vegetables are also rajasic. Tamasic foods induce lethargy and dull the senses, causing negative emotions. These include red meat, alcohol, and mushrooms.

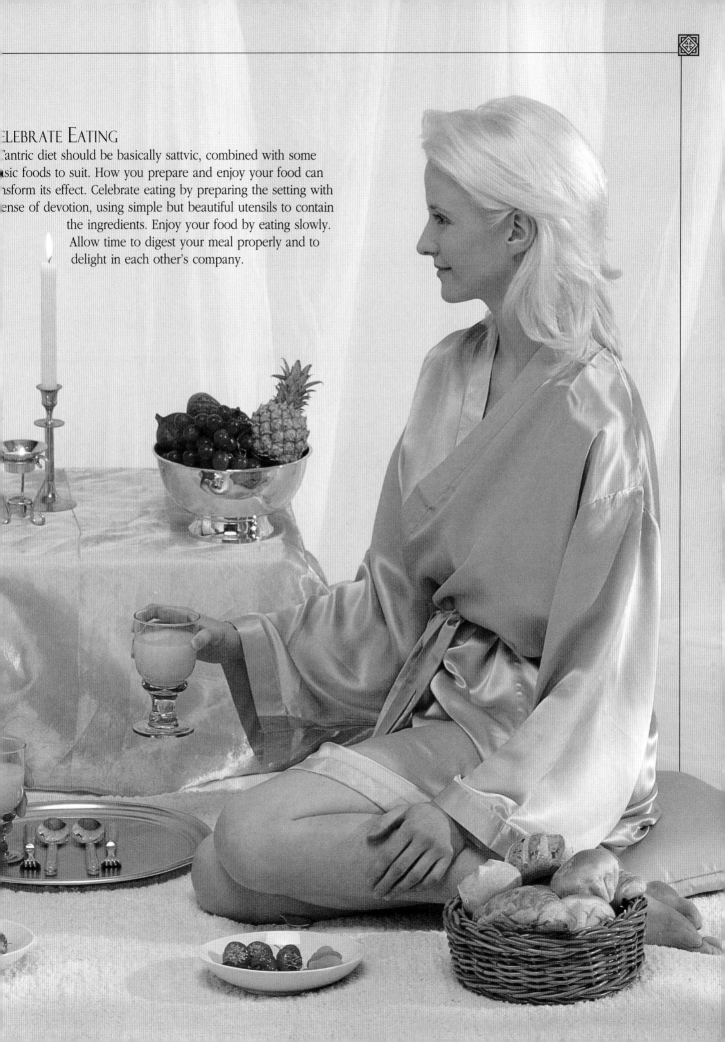

CELEBRATE EATING

A Tantric diet should be basically sattvic, combined with some rajasic foods to suit. How you prepare and enjoy your food can transform its effect. Celebrate eating by preparing the setting with a sense of devotion, using simple but beautiful utensils to contain the ingredients. Enjoy your food by eating slowly. Allow time to digest your meal properly and to delight in each other's company.

YOGIC PRANAYAMA

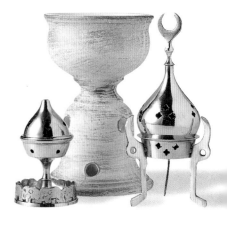

PRANAYAMA is the conscious regulation of breath that is fundamental to all Tantric practices. By controlling the breath, and bringing it into a fuller and more harmonious rhythmic pattern, you are able to master body, mind, and emotions. Breath is the vehicle of prana, which is the very essence of universal life energy. Prana exists in all things, whether manifested or unmanifested. It is the link between the physical and etheric body, the Self and Existence. Consciously circulated within you, prana enhances vitality and self-awareness. It also accelerates the practitioner's spiritual evolution by awakening dormant Kundalini or Shakti energy, enabling it to rise through the subtle body channels.

PRANIC AROMAS
Certain incenses or aromatic oils can help you to concentrate your mind and elevate your spirit during pranayama practice. Frankincense, sandalwood, and cedarwood have all been used traditionally to enhance pranayama, meditation, and worship.

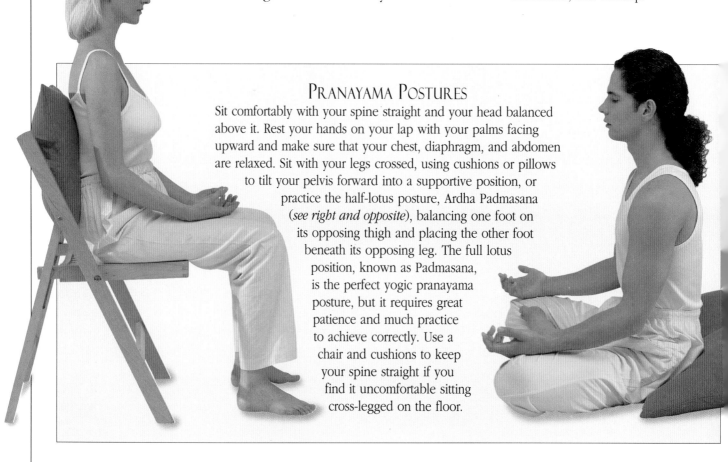

PRANAYAMA POSTURES
Sit comfortably with your spine straight and your head balanced above it. Rest your hands on your lap with your palms facing upward and make sure that your chest, diaphragm, and abdomen are relaxed. Sit with your legs crossed, using cushions or pillows to tilt your pelvis forward into a supportive position, or practice the half-lotus posture, Ardha Padmasana (*see right and opposite*), balancing one foot on its opposing thigh and placing the other foot beneath its opposing leg. The full lotus position, known as Padmasana, is the perfect yogic pranayama posture, but it requires great patience and much practice to achieve correctly. Use a chair and cushions to keep your spine straight if you find it uncomfortable sitting cross-legged on the floor.

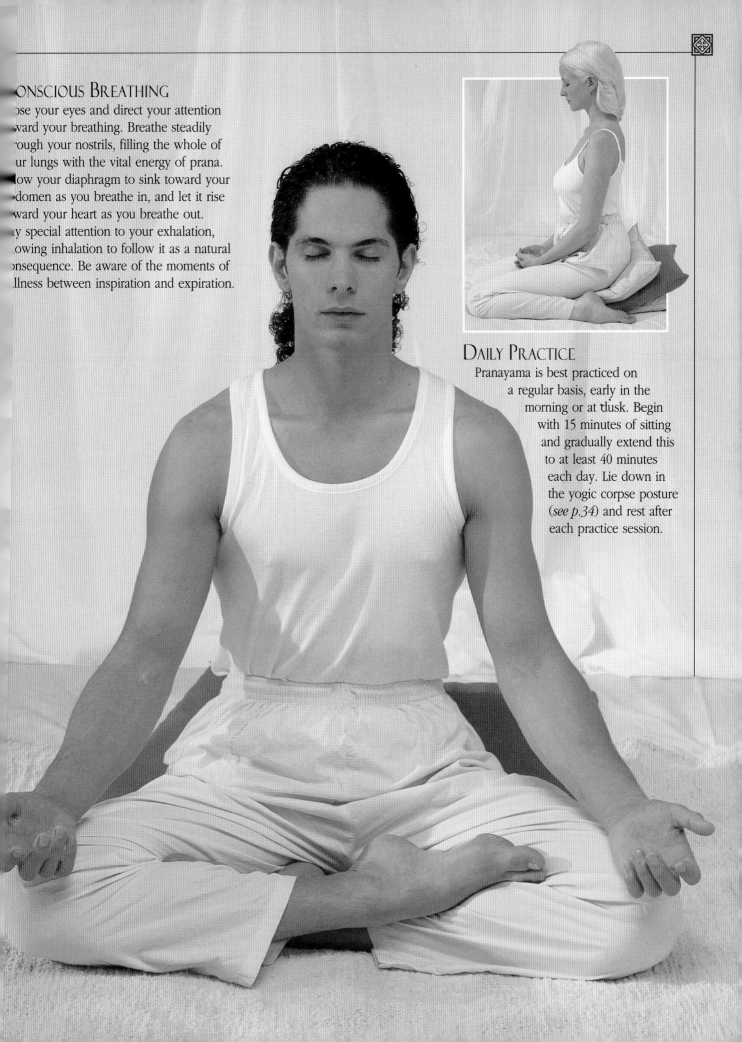

CONSCIOUS BREATHING

Close your eyes and direct your attention toward your breathing. Breathe steadily through your nostrils, filling the whole of your lungs with the vital energy of prana. Allow your diaphragm to sink toward your abdomen as you breathe in, and let it rise toward your heart as you breathe out. Pay special attention to your exhalation, allowing inhalation to follow it as a natural consequence. Be aware of the moments of stillness between inspiration and expiration.

DAILY PRACTICE

Pranayama is best practiced on a regular basis, early in the morning or at dusk. Begin with 15 minutes of sitting and gradually extend this to at least 40 minutes each day. Lie down in the yogic corpse posture (*see p.34*) and rest after each practice session.

HARNESSING BREATH

ACCORDING TO TANTRA, the same polar energies that govern the laws of the cosmos also exist within us. The advanced pranayama technique described here balances the solar and lunar psychic forces flowing through the energy channels, or nadis, that pervade the subtle body (*see p.12*). Breathing alternately through the left and right nostrils purifies and balances Ida and Pingala – the two main nadis entwined around the central energy channel, Sushumna, along which the Kundalini energy rises. Ida, which is connected to the left nostril, represents white, feminine, moon energy; Pingala, which is connected to the right nostril, represents red, masculine, sun energy. Practice the Single Nostril Breathing (*see right*) before proceeding to the more advanced second exercise. Repeat each exercise at least ten times.

"Prana, the *vital breath*, is born of the Self." PRANA UPANISHAD

HAND MUDRA
Use this hand position, known as a mudra, to close one nostril at a time or to seal off both while retaining the breath. Alternate Nostril Breathing regulates the three phases of a breath cycle – inspiration, retention, and expiration – to a ratio of 1:4:2.

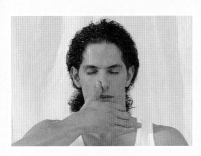
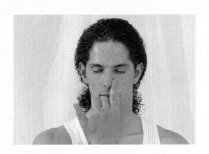

SINGLE NOSTRIL BREATHING

First press your thumb against your right nostril. Inhale through your left nostril to a count of four. Breathe out to a count of eight. Then press the ring and little finger against the left nostril, inhaling for a count of four through the right nostril. Exhale to a count of eight.

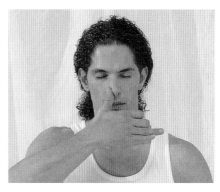

STAGE 1

Begin this Alternate Nostril Breathing exercise by pressing your thumb firmly against your right nostril. Inhale evenly through the left nostril to a count of two.

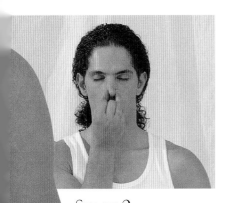

STAGE 2

Pinch both nostrils closed by adding pressure on the left nostril from the ring and little fingers and retain your breath for a count of eight.

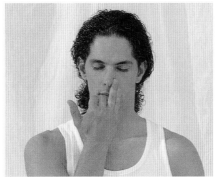

STAGE 3

Release the pressure of the thumb and breathe out steadily through your right nostril for a count of four to complete the required breathing ratio of 1:4:2.

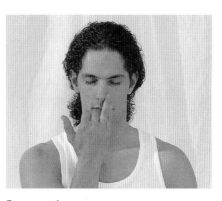

STAGE 4

For the next phase of the breathing cycle, keep your two fingers pressed against your left nostril and inhale for a count of two through your right nostril.

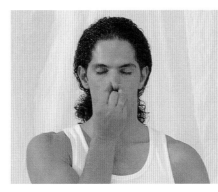

STAGE 5

Now, once again, close up both nostrils by sealing the right nostril by applying a firm pressure with your thumb, and retain your breath for a count of eight.

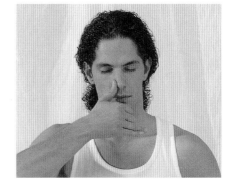

STAGE 6

To complete a whole cycle of Alternate Nostril Breathing, exhale through your left nostril for a count of four. Repeat the breath cycle at least ten times.

MEDITATING TOGETHER

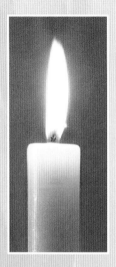

MEDITATION INSTILLS CALM and focus into your lives. If you and your partner meditate together on a regular basis, then you are making a mutual commitment to engender greater awareness and spiritual growth within your relationship. Meditation has always been a major tool for Tantric disciples in their search for enlightenment. It can help you to know and understand yourself better, while deepening your sense of connection to the cosmic whole. It will teach you to be more in the moment and less in the mind, and will therefore bring a more meditative quality to your love life. To meditate, wear simple and comfortable clothing. Create a tranquil environment, and adorn your shrine with lighted candles, incense, and other objects that help you to focus your mind.

"I *bow to Thee*, who in His Essence is One, and who grants *Liberation*." MAHANIRVANA TANTRA

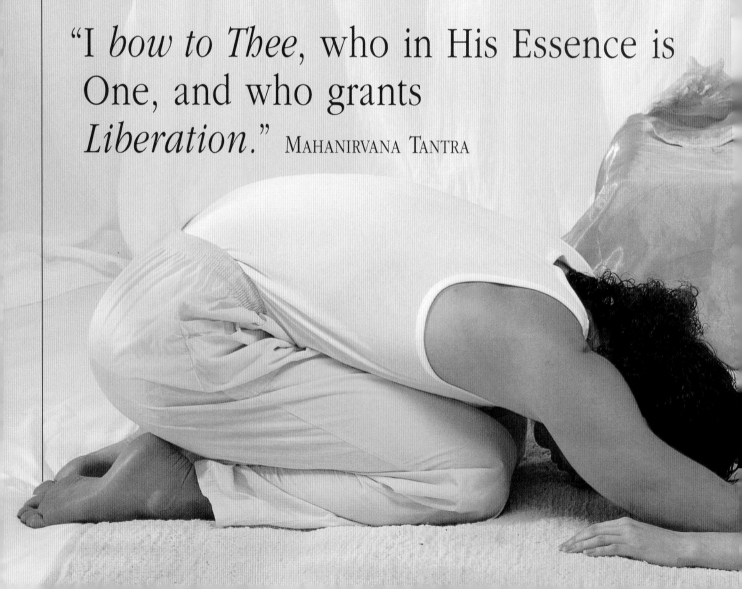

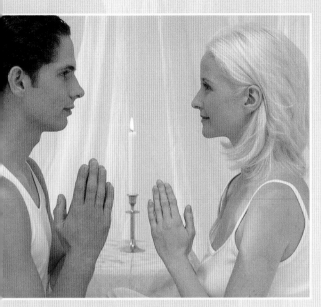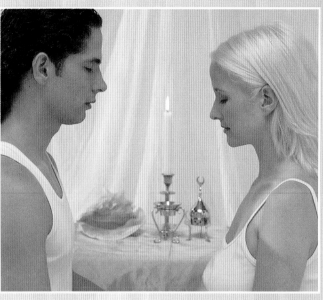

GREETING THE DIVINE

A beautiful way to begin and end each meditation sitting is to use the Hindu gesture of greeting, Namaste, where the hands are raised to the heart in the prayer position. Through this auspicious gesture, you honor the divinity within your Tantric partner and in yourself, and you acknowledge the sanctity of the situation.

SITTING SILENTLY

Assume the position taken for pranayama (*see p.102*). Close your eyes, allowing your thoughts to come and go. Focus your awareness onto the rise and fall of your abdomen as you inhale and exhale. When your attention wanders, bring it back to your breath. Meditate for 15 minutes initially, and gradually extend this period to 40 to 60 minutes per session.

GRATITUDE & GRACE

After meditating, surrender yourselves to the feelings of oneness that can fill you with a profound sense of gratitude and grace. Bow down to the earth in a supine posture of prayer, as shown below, or relax in the corpse posture with your back flat against the floor. Then take time to rest and assimilate your experiences before resuming normal activities.

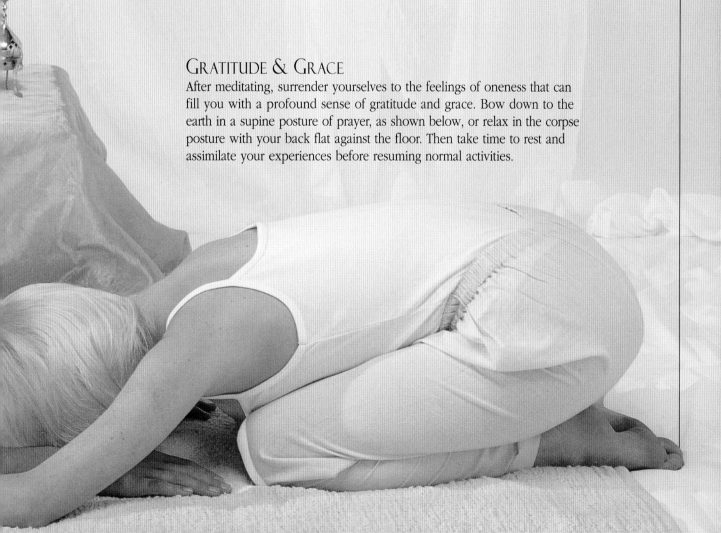

FOCUSING THE MIND

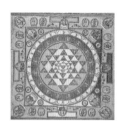

ONCE MEDITATION PRACTICE has become a regular part of your relationship, you will realize just how easily the mind is distracted. The purpose of meditation is to still the mind but not to repress it. Tantrikas have many techniques to aid meditation, but the principle of all meditation rituals is to focus the mind on a single point, whether through awareness, sight, or sound. Yantras, such as the Shri Yantra shown above, are powerful visual aids for concentration. Whenever your mind wanders, which will be frequently for the novice, you gently bring your attention back to the point of focus at the center of the geometric pattern. Practice the following techniques in your sacred space, alone or with your partner, to increase the potency of your contemplation. In time, the essence of meditation will arise within you like a benediction.

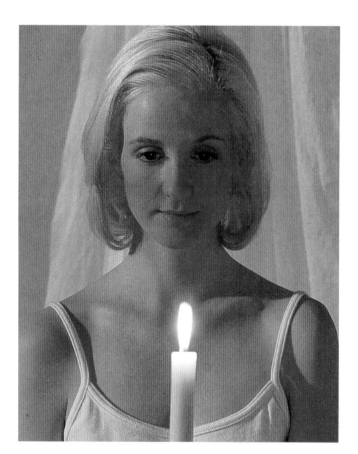

"When the *breath* is steady..., so is the *mind*..."

HATHA YOGA PRADIPIKA

CANDLE GAZING

Tratak meditation uses an external visual object as a focal point of stillness. As such, the steady flame of a candle is the perfect tool. Place a lighted candle, at eye level, about one meter away from you. Gaze softly and steadily at the flame without blinking and until your eyes begin to water. Then close your eyes and hold the mental vision of the flame. When the image fades, return your vision to the external flame. Repeat the process for up to 40 minutes.

HUMMING MEDITATION

Repeating a special vibratory sound, known as a mantra, is another technique for quietening the wandering nature of the mind. You can begin to explore the potent effect of sound vibration by humming. Start to hum so that it resonates from deep within your body, reverberating through the chakras and then out into the environment. You will soon discover your own natural tone and pitch. Practice alone or with your partner until you can hum together for 40 minutes.

THE OM SYMBOL

Placed on your altar, the Om symbol is the ideal focal point for contemplation – as is its repeated intonation as a mantra. According to ancient Hindu scriptures, it represents the source from which the Supreme Consciousness emanates. The Om mantra, pronounced as A-U-M, is the primordial sound, the sacred syllable, the ultimate vibration, which created the universe and symbolizes a state of perfect equilibrium and harmonious union.

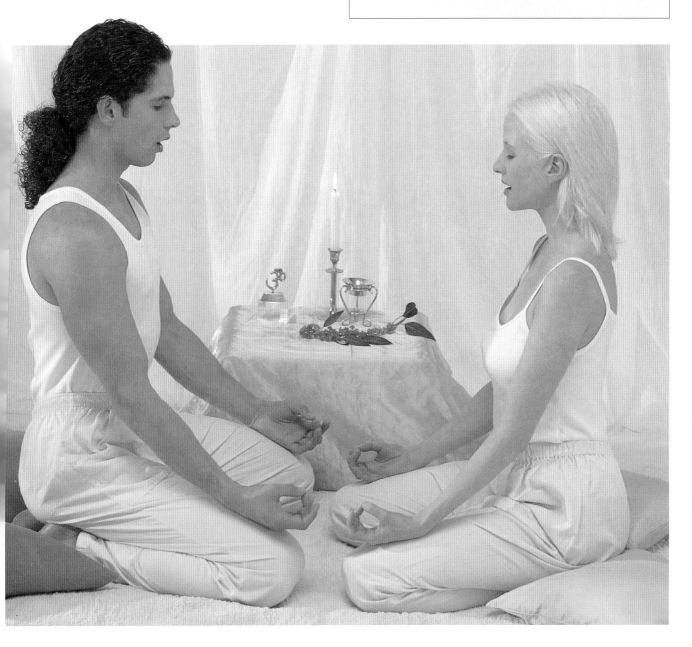

CHAKRA BREATHING

BY SENDING HEALING BREATH into each of the seven main energy chakras, and by connecting more deeply to these vortice of cosmic power within you, you begin to open windows to th Divine and become more attuned to your inner sense of Self. Start by absorbing the information relating to chakras in the introduction to this book, noting particularly the specific spiritual significance and location within the subtle body of each chakra. Begin the exercises by using a visualizatio technique to purify the Kundalini pathway, which is the abode of the seven energy chakras (*see left*). As you inhale imagine that you are drawing a golden light in through the crown chakra. Exhale, sending the light, breath by breath, down through the spine toward the base chakra. Always rest for five or six minutes after chakra meditation before resuming normal activities.

CHAKRA VISUALIZATION

To stimulate each chakra individually, direct your awareness toward each energy center for about three minutes in turn. Start at the base chakra and move upward to the crown chakra. Visualize a radiant light within each energy center. The light's hue should correspond to the color related to the individual chakra (*see above*). Each inhalation strengthens the purity of the color, and each exhalation expands its luminosity. Complete the meditation by imagining a cleansing golden light sweeping down the Sushumna.

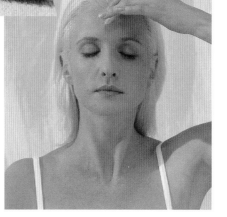
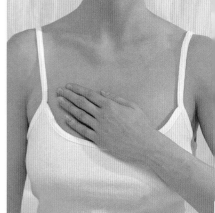

BEING IN TOUCH

When meditating on individual chakras, it often helps to touch its location to strengthen its connection to your physical body. For example, touch the center of your forehead when focusing on the third eye chakra, and touch the center of your chest when focusing on the heart chakra.

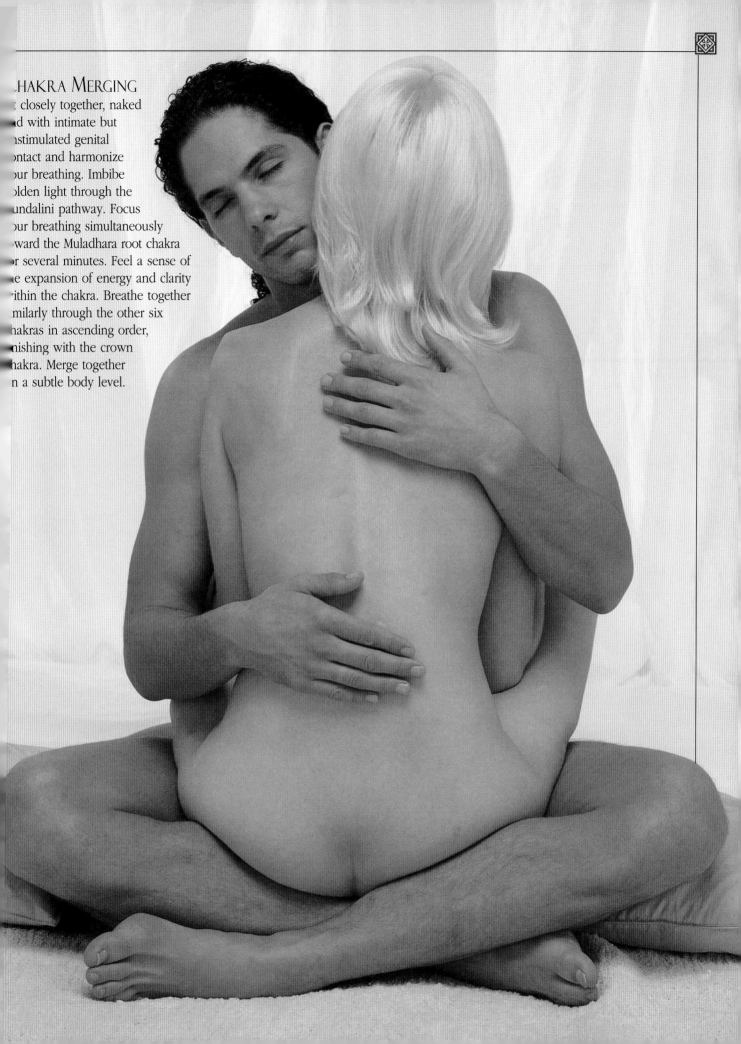

CHAKRA MERGING

...t closely together, naked
...d with intimate but
...nstimulated genital
...ntact and harmonize
...ur breathing. Imbibe
...olden light through the
...undalini pathway. Focus
...ur breathing simultaneously
...ward the Muladhara root chakra
...r several minutes. Feel a sense of
...e expansion of energy and clarity
...ithin the chakra. Breathe together
...milarly through the other six
...hakras in ascending order,
...nishing with the crown
...hakra. Merge together
...n a subtle body level.

CLEANSING THE HEART

THE HEART CHAKRA is the energetic center for integration and merging. When it is open, we want to dissolve ourselves with the beloved other, whether that is represented by a lover or by the sense of the Divine. According to Tantric teachings, it is in the heart chakra that the physical and psychic realities meet and where there is union between feminine and masculine energies. Cleansing the heart through meditation helps to heal old hurts, so that you are able to share your love unconditionally and be more empathetic with others. The following meditations will help this process to unfold. Spend up to 15 minutes on each, using them separately or combining them so that the love-channeling follows the eye-gazing exercise.

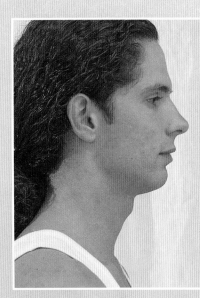

EYE CONTACT
Create a circuit of energy between you by placing your right palm on the upturned left hand of your partner. Breathe steadily, and relax your faces. Look deeply but softly into each other's eyes, revealing your essential selves. See and be seen to the core of your hearts. Then close your eyes and spend a few moments longer focusing your attention inward. Allow feelings to arise without attempting to control them.

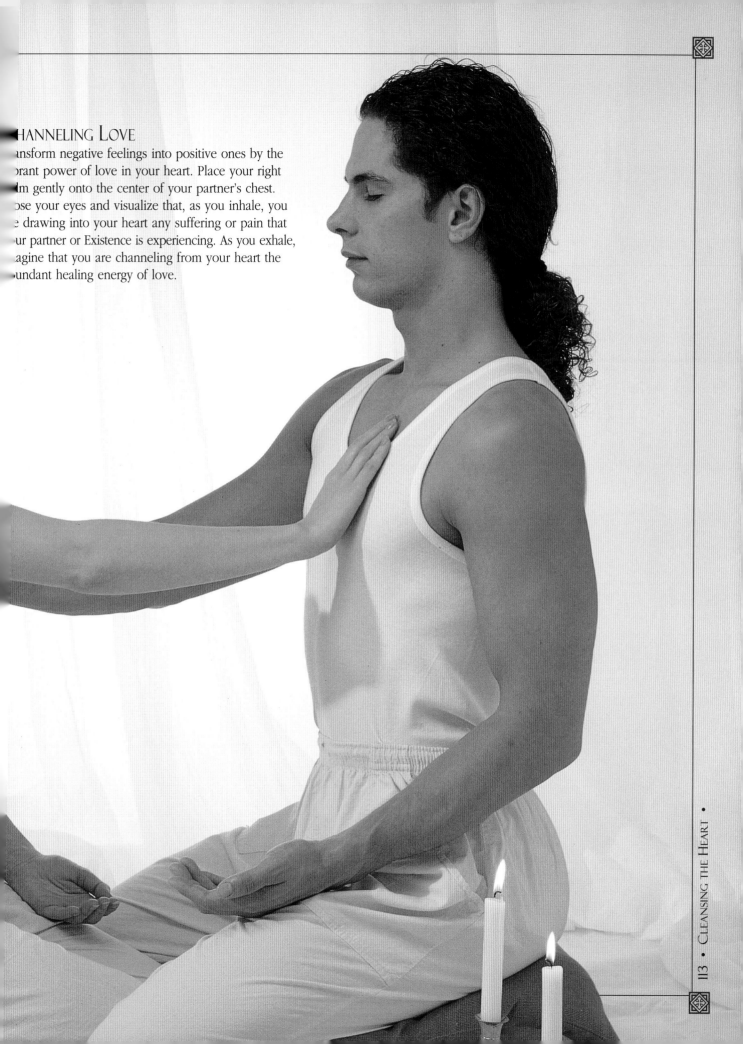

CHANNELING LOVE

Transform negative feelings into positive ones by the vibrant power of love in your heart. Place your right palm gently onto the center of your partner's chest. Close your eyes and visualize that, as you inhale, you are drawing into your heart any suffering or pain that your partner or Existence is experiencing. As you exhale, imagine that you are channeling from your heart the abundant healing energy of love.

THE ENERGY BODY

YOU ARE pure energy. It pulsates through you, creating your physical vitality, your mental thoughts, your emotions, your love, and your potential for bliss. Energy at its rawest is sexual; energy at its most refined is spiritual. But all energy emanates from the one cosmic source. The more you experience yourself as energy, the more connected you feel with existence. By becoming increasingly sensitive toward the movement of energy within and all around you, you tap into the subtler and more metaphysical level of your being, bringing a transcendental quality to your meditation and lovemaking.

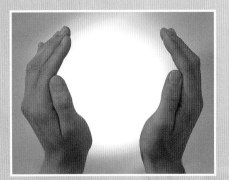

FEELING ENERGY
Create an energy field between your own hands or between your hands and those of your partner. Breathe in deeply and steadily, consciously directing the exhalation toward your hands. Visualize this outflow of breath as heat, vibration, or light. Allow a magnetic charge to build up between your palms. Soon you will experience it as a tangible force.

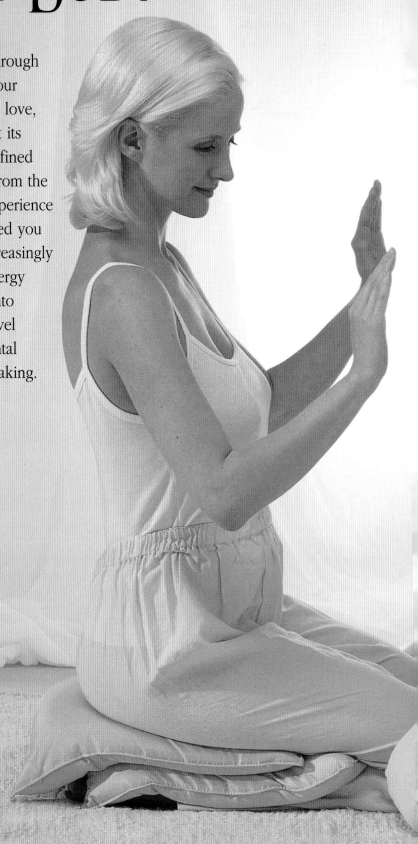

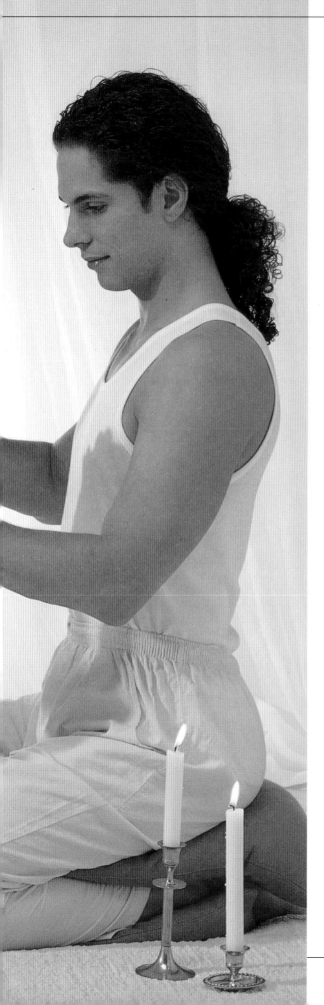

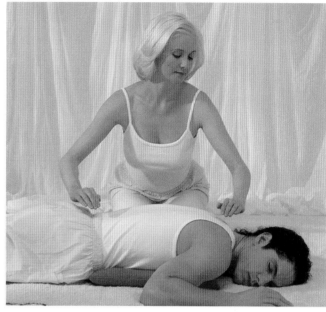

LOVING INTENTION

Use your hands to send healing energy toward your lover's spine. Your loving intention, and the heat radiating from your hands, will help to unlock tension and release energy blocks from the Kundalini pathway. Move your hands over different areas of the spine when you feel intuitively directed to do so.

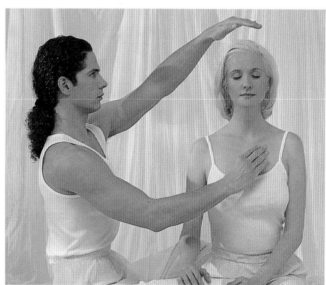

SENSING THE AURA

Move your hands slowly around your partner's body to sense the presence of her aura. Keep your palms open and relaxed, a short distance from her skin. You may experience the aura as a feeling of heat, density, light, tingling, or in visual images and color. These physical sensations may vary from one area to another, particularly when you are closer to the chakras.

TANTRIC MASSAGE

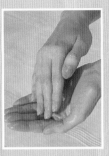

TOUCH is the language of love. During a Tantric massage, your hands connect with the physical, the emotional, and the spiritual levels of your beloved. Through your tactile contact, dissolve yourself into his energy as if you are communicating with his heart and soul. Massage is the perfect medium for realizing that giving and receiving is a reciprocal cycle of energy. Honor and respect your partner's body. Never use massage to manipulate a sexual situation. However, if there is mutual consent, the occasion can become an exquisite prelude to lovemaking.

MASSAGE SPACE

Create a meditative environment in which to massage; this will help you to remain calm and focused and your partner to feel protected and relaxed. Use low, soft lighting, or candlelight, and make sure that the room is warm and draft free. A mattress, or folded-up blankets placed on the floor, provides a more supportive base than the bed. Have a supply of clean sheets and towels for cover and warmth, and use cushions and pillows for comfort and support.

AROMATIC INFLUENCE

Aromatic essential oils enhance the effects of a Tantric massage. For a whole-body massage, blend recommended amounts of oil essences into a basic mix of 25 ml of vegetable oil such as jobobo, almond, or sunflower. The following recipe heightens feelings of sensuality, meditation, and love: six drops of rose absolute, four drops of sandalwood, and five drops of frankincense. Warm the oil between your hands before applying to the skin in smooth, flowing strokes.

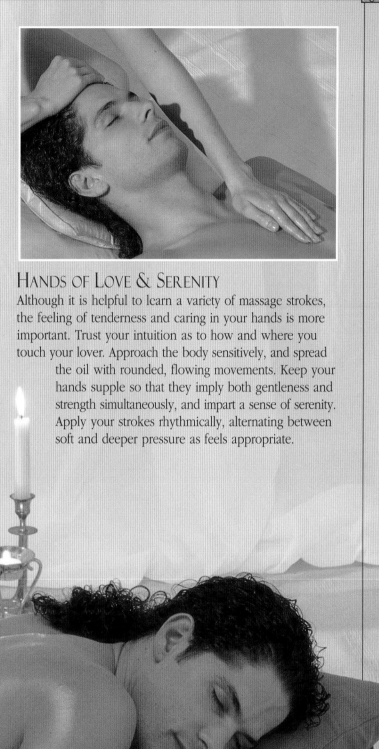

HANDS OF LOVE & SERENITY

Although it is helpful to learn a variety of massage strokes, the feeling of tenderness and caring in your hands is more important. Trust your intuition as to how and where you touch your lover. Approach the body sensitively, and spread the oil with rounded, flowing movements. Keep your hands supple so that they imply both gentleness and strength simultaneously, and impart a sense of serenity. Apply your strokes rhythmically, alternating between soft and deeper pressure as feels appropriate.

"Be in your fingers and hands as
your *whole being, you*
whole soul, is there.

OSHO

PERSONAL TOUCH

Touch your lover's face with reverence
for this is a very personal part of her
body. Applying a small amount of oil,
use steady and reassuring strokes that
define her features and soothe away
her cares. Make small, flowing fingertip
circles over her cheeks and around her
chin. Glide your hands up over her neck
and head to draw tension away from her.

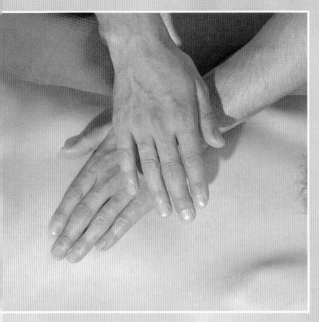

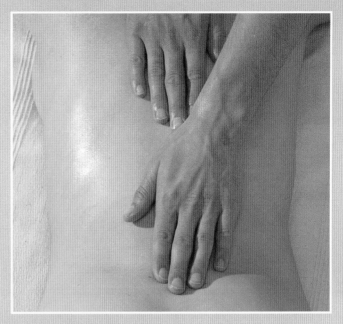

EDIUM OF TRUST

oke the soft round mound of the abdomen in circular
:ions to relax emotional and physical tensions that can
bit the flow of sexual and vital energy. Approach this
herable area with awareness, letting your touch be the
dium through which trust deepens between you.

FOCUS ON SPINE

A flexible spine enables the Kundalini energy to rise during
meditation and lovemaking. Relax the spine by gliding your
hands down each side several times. Use shorter but deeper
grinding movements from thumbs and fingers to release
tightness closer to the bone.

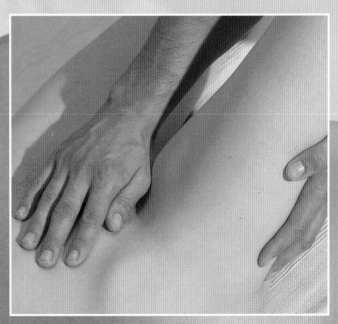

GENITAL TOUCH

With clear consent from your receptive partner, you can
apply loving strokes on and around the genital area. The
sincerity and warmth of your touch will ensure that these
intimate parts feel more sensual and integrated with the
entire body, enhancing emotional and sexual relaxation.

TANTRIC SEXUALITY

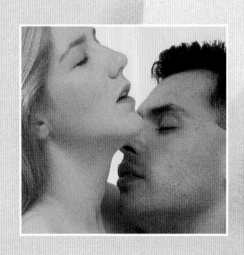

"By concentrating the ecstatic forces within, wonderful visions dawn in the mind's eye. This is a special secret, which shortens the journey to Liberation"

YOGINI TANTRA

IF YOU ARE ABLE TO MAKE LOVE WITHOUT INVOLVING YOUR EGOS, AND WITHOUT PRESSURE OR expectation, you can transform your sexuality into something

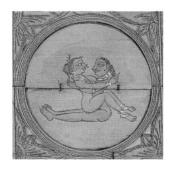

This painting depicts a Tantric couple copulating in the high sex seated posture used in mystical sex rituals.

that is blissful and transcendental. Give yourself totally and unconditionally to your Tantric lover, and you will liberate your ECSTATIC *spirit*. Allow your lovemaking to become a moment to moment experience, unconcerned with the pursuit of orgasm as the ultimate goal, and you will attain a TIMELESS *quality,* a blissful sense of oneness with your beloved.

TO HARNESS the full potential of your sexuality you must bring a profound commitment to your lovemaking and understand that your pursuit of TRUE *sexual happiness* is inextricably linked to the pursuit of spiritual fulfillment. Bring a SENSE *of sacredness* to all your lovemaking. Even simply lying together in conjugal unity, breathing synchronistically, making eye contact, and being silent together for just 15 minutes can be part of your Tantric sex. Or you may make love for many hours, even many days, because you can leave each other's side and return later to continue your extended sexual intercourse, creating and CHANNELING *orgasmic energy.*

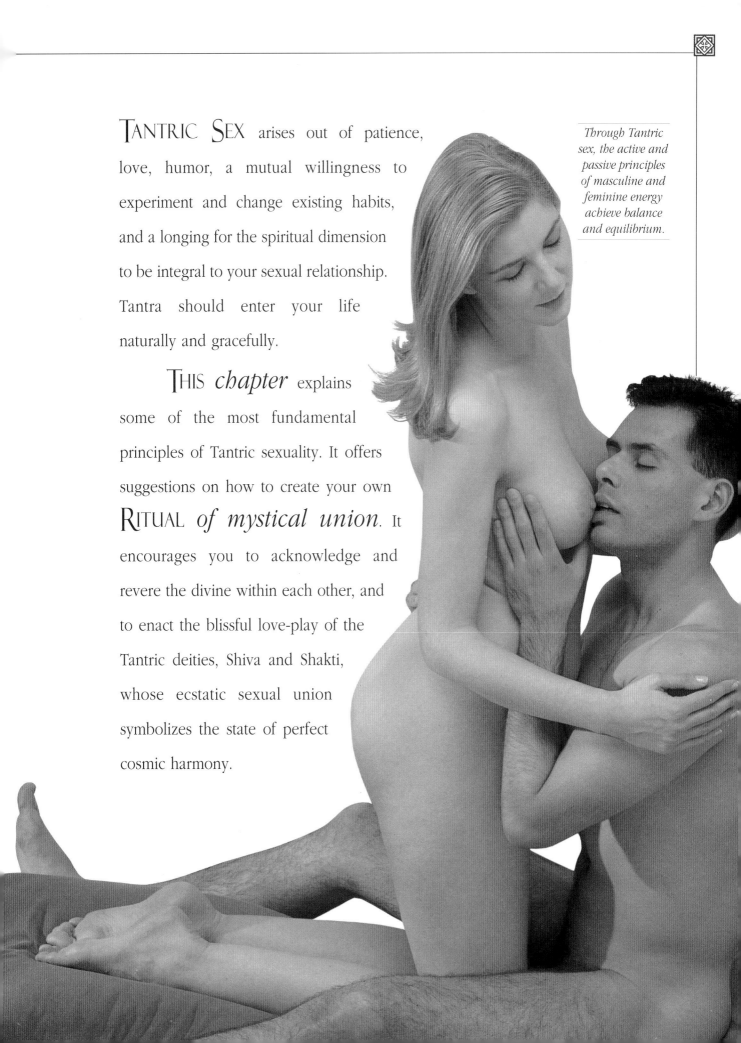

TANTRIC SEX arises out of patience, love, humor, a mutual willingness to experiment and change existing habits, and a longing for the spiritual dimension to be integral to your sexual relationship. Tantra should enter your life naturally and gracefully.

THIS *chapter* explains some of the most fundamental principles of Tantric sexuality. It offers suggestions on how to create your own RITUAL *of mystical union*. It encourages you to acknowledge and revere the divine within each other, and to enact the blissful love-play of the Tantric deities, Shiva and Shakti, whose ecstatic sexual union symbolizes the state of perfect cosmic harmony.

Through Tantric sex, the active and passive principles of masculine and feminine energy achieve balance and equilibrium.

THE SEED OF LIFE

TANTRA TEACHES A MAN to gain control over his normally involuntary ejaculation process so that the potent life-force energy of his semen is channeled toward sexual and spiritual ecstasy. Through Tantra, and with love, patience, and humor, you can learn to retain your semen and prolong lovemaking. Ejaculation often leads to energy depletion for the man, and consequent sexual dissatisfaction for the woman. Tantra teaches you to contain your sexual excitement by steadying your thoughts and focusing your breath. It encourages the man to learn to recognize when he is approaching the heightened arousal state prior to ejaculatory inevitability, and teaches him to slow down at this plateau stage.

STAY RELAXED
Both partners must become mindful of their own and their partner's sexual responses, approaching sex meditatively and with less excitement. Positions where the man is relaxed, such as when the woman is on top or when the couple lie side by side facing each other, can help prolong lovemaking.

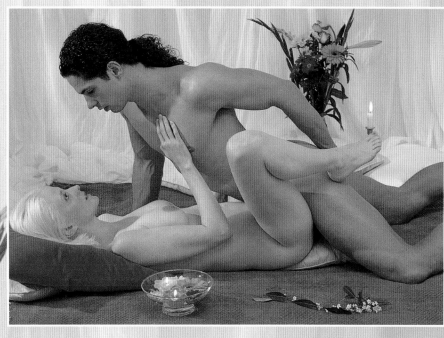

PRESSURE POINT

A Tantric technique for preventing imminent ejaculation is to apply firm fingertip pressure to a perineum point between the anus and the scrotum. At the same time you should steady your breath and still your mind. The pressure can prevent semen from leaving the prostate gland, though you may still be able to experience the pleasurable involuntary contractions associated with orgasm.

MALE SELF-PLEASURING

Practice this exercise alone to gain more control over your pre-orgasmic responses. Stroke each part of your body erotically, including your sexual organs. As orgasmic sensations increase, relax your pelvic floor muscles and, breathing steadily, imagine those pleasurable feelings spreading away from the genital area and flooding across your whole body.

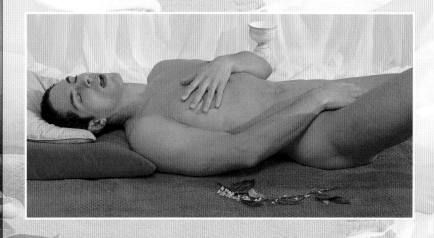

PLATEAU OF LOVE

IF EXCITEMENT, passion, and fantasy have been the main ingredients of your sexual relationship, then Tantric sex may seem a little cool at first. This feeling will last only until you gain the ability to surrender yourselves wholly and spontaneously into your sexual communion. Focus your awareness onto each sensation as it arises and return to that present moment of experience when the urge is there to rush headlong toward orgasm. Be less cerebral and more physically attuned to each other, breathing together and keeping eye contact. Relish the more subtle delights of the plateau phase of lovemaking.

"Do not eject semen *casually*. ... Its nature is *supreme joy*." HEVAJRA TANTRA

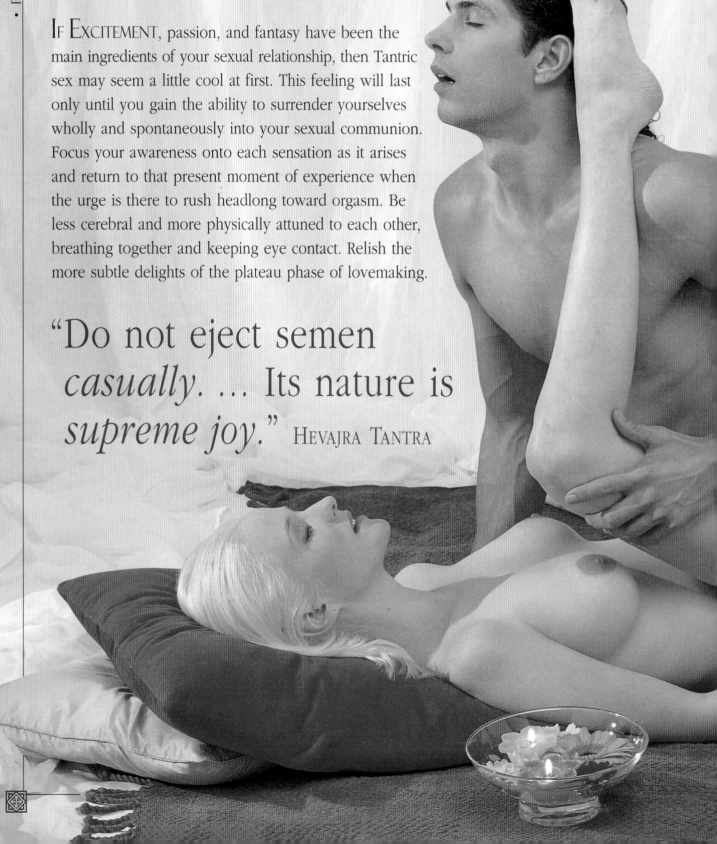

ANTRIC TECHNIQUE

sexual excitement reaches a critical
ase and you approach the brink of
gasm, stop moving. Relax together,
bmerging yourselves into a feeling
mutual stillness. A Tantric technique
vises the man to press his tongue
mly onto the roof of his mouth
hile steadying his thoughts and
eath to avoid semen ejaculation.

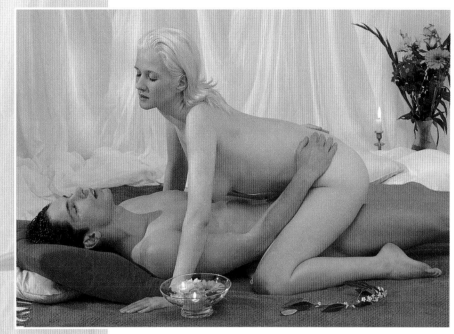

FEMALE ORGASM

Many women are filled with a renewed vitality after orgasm,
while others are multiorgasmic. Some women, however, feel
as depleted as their partners after orgasm. In this case, the
female partner should also contain her orgasmic energy,
allowing it to build up rather than dissipating it, and she
should slow her movements down if she is overaroused.

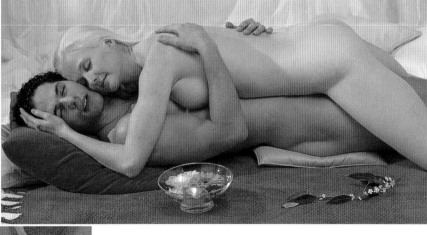

BODY TO BODY

It is not necessary for the man's penis to remain fully erect
at all times. Relax together at times, body to body, moving
only enough to arouse the penis sufficiently for the sexual
contact to be maintained. In your stillness, feel as if all the
physical boundaries between you are slowly melting away.

CIRCULATING ENERGY

MAKING LOVE is potentially a dance of two energies rather than a physical meeting of two bodies. The natural motions of sex – movement, deep breathing, sighs, sounds, smells, and touch – generate and intensify the subtle but potent energies within you. Tantric lovemaking positions harness and contain these energies within the body so they are not unnecessarily wasted or leaked. Use breath awareness and visualization to consciously circulate this energy between you. Through its transmission, you begin to dissolve the duality of your male and female sexualities. Feel as if you are two halves of one phenomenon merging back together. By fusing with your external lover, you harmonize and balance your own inner masculine and feminine polar energies. Through this internal integration, you can attain a sense of oneness with existence.

"As is the *goddess,* so also is Shiva. They are as the Moon and the *moonlight...*" SHIVA PURANA

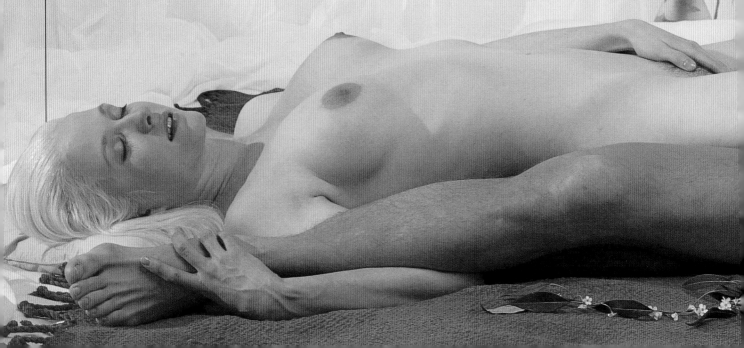

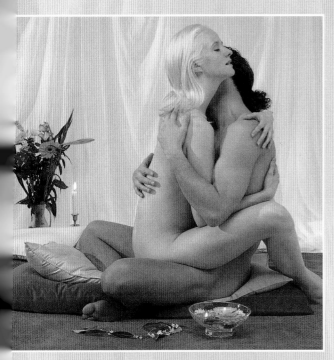

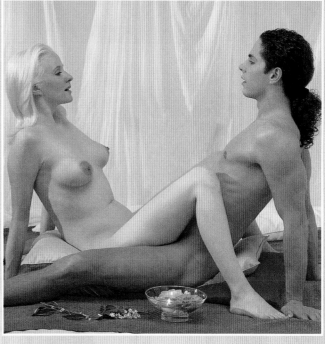

EATED POSTURE

he seated lovemaking position is a principal Tantric sexual
osture. Shakti energy is sealed into the body because the
enitals are interlocked, and the extended spine enhances
s flow through subtle energy channels. Entwined heart to
eart, sway gently together, circulating feelings of love.

LEANING BACK

From the seated position, lean back and maintain eye contact.
Generate Shakti energy with subtle pelvic rocking motions,
contracting your pelvic floor muscles. Use your breath and
visualize your energies streaming upward to merge above
your heads before showering radiant light down upon you.

MANDALA OF LOVE

Trust your body's impulses to take you spontaneously from one
position to another and from activity to rest. Relax awhile, but
remain co-joined. Lie with your spines extended and your yoni
and lingam united. Clasp each other's feet so that your bodies
form a mandala and become a natural wheel of circulating energy.

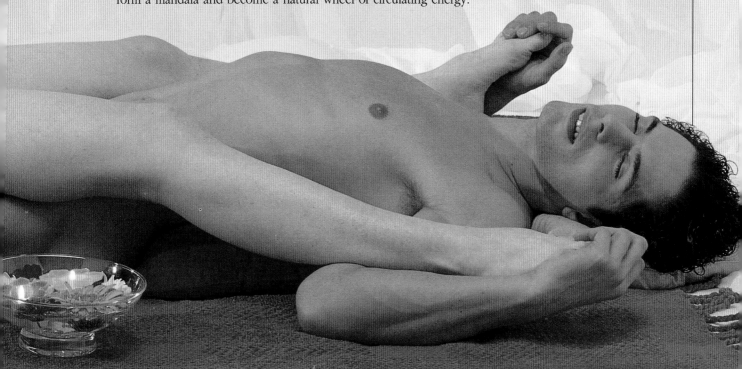

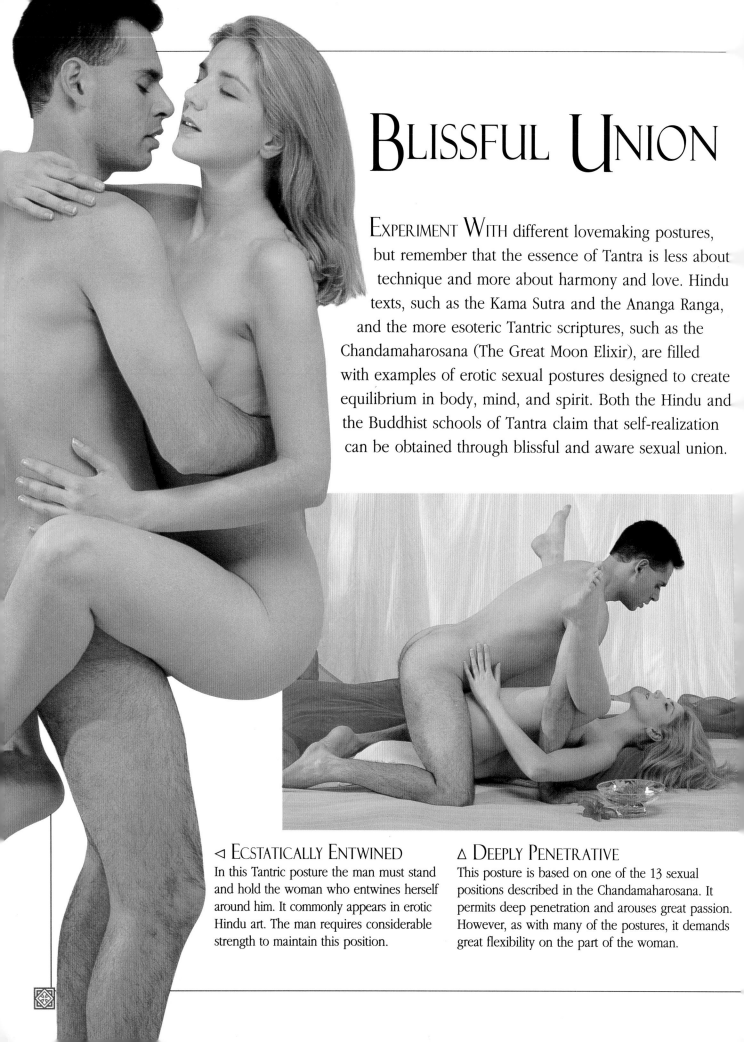

BLISSFUL UNION

EXPERIMENT WITH different lovemaking postures, but remember that the essence of Tantra is less about technique and more about harmony and love. Hindu texts, such as the Kama Sutra and the Ananga Ranga, and the more esoteric Tantric scriptures, such as the Chandamaharosana (The Great Moon Elixir), are filled with examples of erotic sexual postures designed to create equilibrium in body, mind, and spirit. Both the Hindu and the Buddhist schools of Tantra claim that self-realization can be obtained through blissful and aware sexual union.

◁ ECSTATICALLY ENTWINED
In this Tantric posture the man must stand and hold the woman who entwines herself around him. It commonly appears in erotic Hindu art. The man requires considerable strength to maintain this position.

△ DEEPLY PENETRATIVE
This posture is based on one of the 13 sexual positions described in the Chandamaharosana. It permits deep penetration and arouses great passion. However, as with many of the postures, it demands great flexibility on the part of the woman.

Different ways of *lovemaking* generate love, friendship, and respect."

KAMA SUTRA

TOTALLY AUSPICIOUS

This lovemaking posture, aptly called Totally Auspicious, is described in the ninth-century scripture, the Chandamaharosana Tantra. It exquisitely captures the essence of Tantra. The man lifts his lover's feet up toward his upper body so that their soles touch him as if in blessing. The man draws his lover's feet up to touch his mouth and forehead. These gestures convey the man's tenderness, humility, and devotion to his partner.

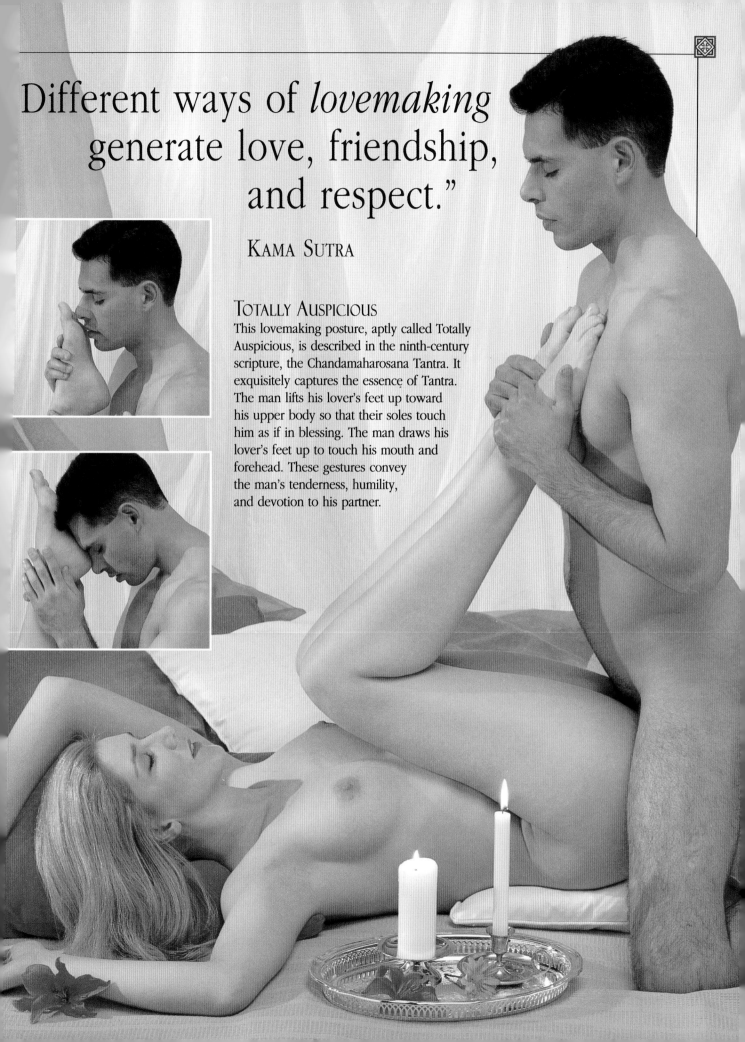

THE NECTAR OF LOVE

EXALT YOUR FEMALE partner when making love to her, because she personifies the essence of the eternal goddess. In Tantra, the woman is perceived as Shakti, the creative cosmic energy. Only through her can the man be initiated into sacred sexual mysteries. When you make love, tell her how much you love her, compliment her, and make her feel she is divine. Tantra understands a woman's potential to be sexually ecstatic and multiorgasmic. It says that female sexual secretions are lotus nectar – the food of the gods. When a woman is sexually fulfilled, her love juices contain magical and restorative properties (*see safe sex guidelines, p.16*).

KALI POWER
Tantrikas considered it very auspicious to have sex with a woman during her menstruation, believing that at this time, her secretions contained the regenerative energies of the powerful goddess, Kali.

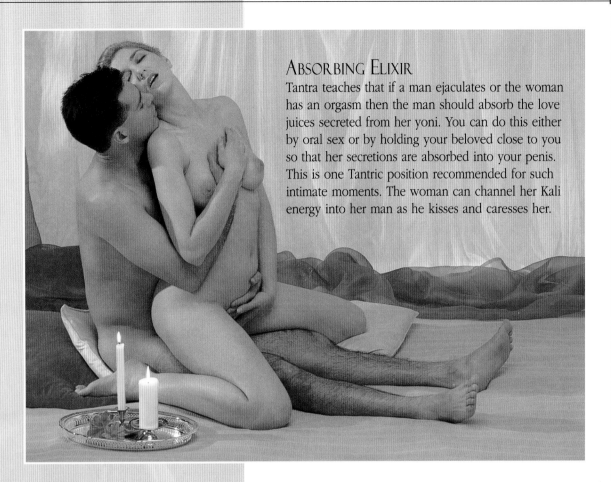

ABSORBING ELIXIR

Tantra teaches that if a man ejaculates or the woman has an orgasm then the man should absorb the love juices secreted from her yoni. You can do this either by oral sex or by holding your beloved close to you so that her secretions are absorbed into your penis. This is one Tantric position recommended for such intimate moments. The woman can channel her Kali energy into her man as he kisses and caresses her.

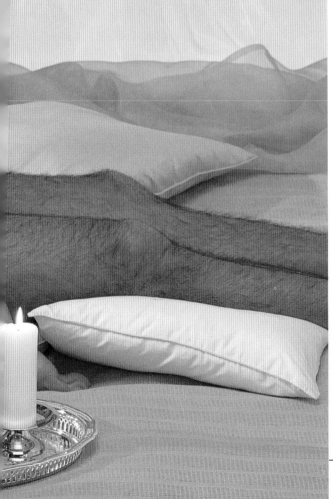

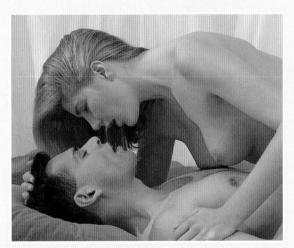

ORGASMIC KISS

When a woman is orgasmic, her saliva is said to contain properties that harmonize the male and female polar energies. Share your sweet nectar with your man by kissing him deeply at this time. Or playfully exchange your saliva, letting it fall like dew drops into his mouth.

RITUALS OF MYSTICAL UNION

TRADITIONAL TANTRIKAS performed elaborate rituals during their mystical sex rites. Each stage of the ceremony, held under the guidance of a spiritually enlightened teacher, was accompanied by stringent personal ablutions; offerings of incense, flowers, and food; recitals of prayers and mantras; and the contemplation of yantras and mandalas. Pranayama techniques and yoga asanas were practiced, and the presence of the Divine Goddess was invoked and worshiped. These rites were carried out in rarefied environments and at auspicious times of the month or day. (The hours between midnight and three in the morning were considered especially significant.) As a modern couple, you must create your own ritual of beliefs and circumstances. Dedicate at least three hours of undisturbed time to the ceremony. The steps shown here are loosely adapted from traditional Tantric rituals. Follow this sequence or create your own, entering each stage with commitment, love, and joy. Let Tantra become not only a method of improving your sex life but also a profound spiritual awakening.

"The phallic and the *embodied image* should be washed with *scented* water." SHIVA PURANA

ACT 1: ALTAR OFFERING

Prepare your sanctuary so that it is sensually beautiful and inviting. Burn incense or aromatic oils to imbue the air with delicate fragrance. Place onto your altar scented flowers and significant offerings dedicated by you to the service of love in whatever way this is meaningful to you.

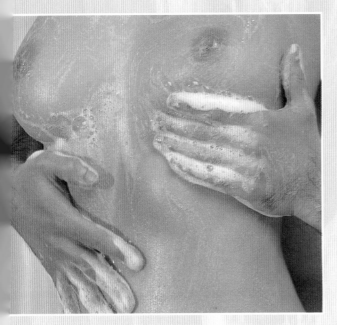

ACT 2: RITUAL BATHING

ght scented candles in your bathroom so it is resplendent
ith a warm glow. Prepare fresh, clean towels ready for use.
ext, ritually bathe each other, allowing the warm water to
ascade over your bodies to wash away all external and
nternal impurities. Then tenderly dry one another.

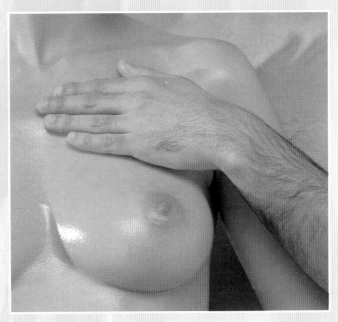

ACT 3: ANOINTING THE WOMAN

The woman should be ritually anointed. Blend a recipe of
uplifting and evocative essential oils with a pure vegetable
oil base, then massage this concoction lovingly all over her
body. Rose, jasmine, sandalwood, ylang-ylang, and neroli
are some appropriate choices of aromatic essences.

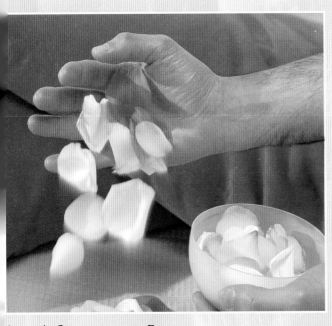

ACT 4: SCATTERING PETALS

Enter your sanctuary together. Bow to each other to honor
the intrinsic divine nature of your partner. Take a bowl of
petals and scatter them about the sanctum to symbolically
consecrate your environment. Place a fragrant flower on the
altar as an offering and invitation to the Higher Spirit of Love.

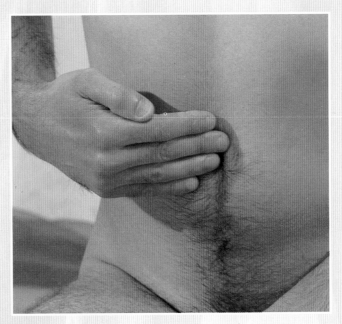

ACT 5: SELF-TOUCH RITUAL

The man can now perform a simple self-touching ceremony
based on the ancient Tantric ritual of nyasa. Touch each part
of your body with the pure intention of letting go of desire
and ego and to consciously sensitize and protect yourself
on a physical- and psychic-body level.

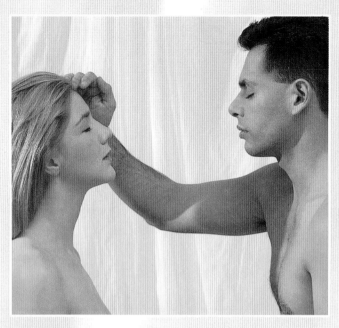

ACT 6: HONORING SHAKTI

Kneeling before your partner, perceive her to be the sacred embodiment of the goddess, Shakti. Touch and honor each part of her body. In Tantric tradition you touch first the left foot, move up her left side to the top of her head, and then back down the other side of her body to her right foot.

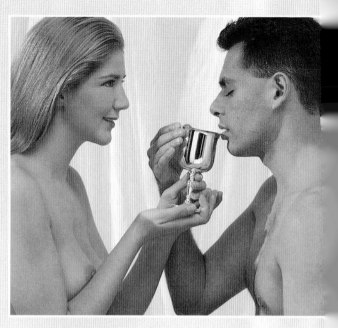

ACT 7: DRINKING WINE

Wine, a forbidden beverage in traditional Hindu culture, was purified by Tantric ritual, as an offering to the deities. Tantric disciples would drink one cup between them, taking turns to sip from the cup with pleasure and awareness. Pour wine (or fruit juice) into a chalice and share it likewise.

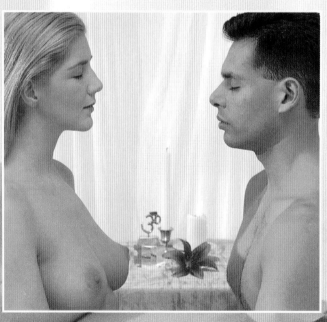

ACT 8: MEDITATION

Play some music that inspires you and your beloved to dance ecstatically together. Become Shiva and Shakti in a dance of creativity and love. Or you may prefer to practice some yoga asanas together. Then sit down and meditate with your lover, steadying your breath and focusing your thoughts.

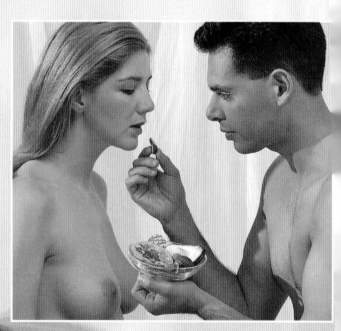

ACT 9: FOOD RITUAL

Before performing their mystical sex rites, Tantrikas partook of a meal of forbidden foods transubstantiated into divine offerings by ritual and prayer. Offer each other morsels of the delicious foods that you have prepared. Allow your sex center to be stimulated by your taste sense.

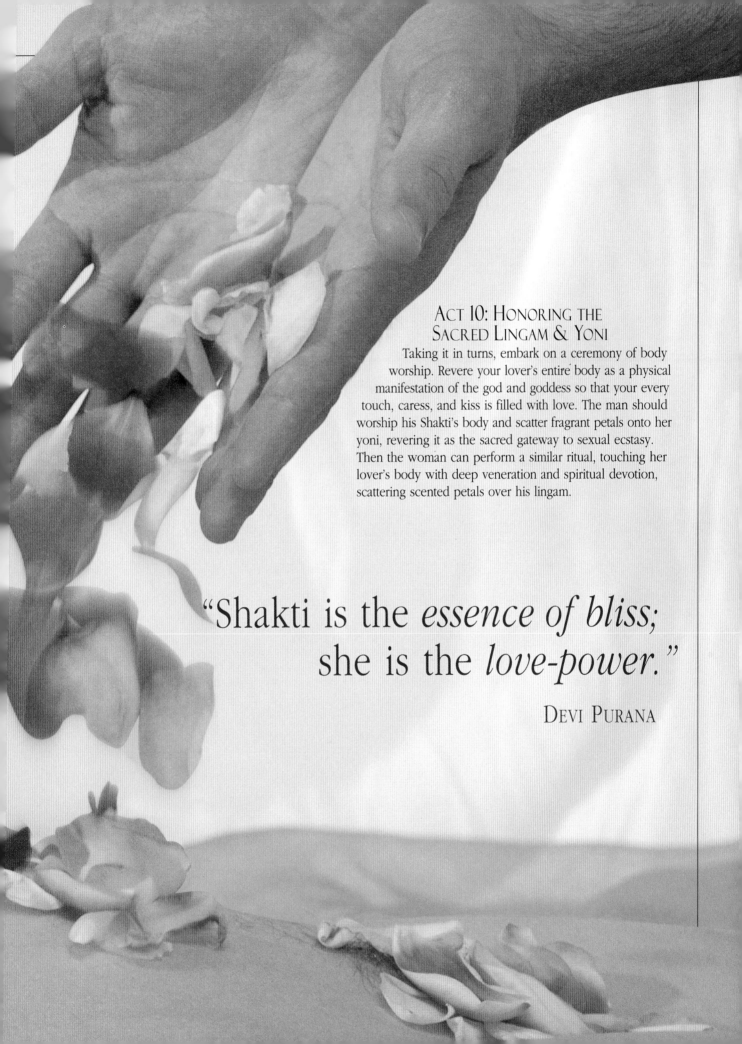

ACT 10: HONORING THE SACRED LINGAM & YONI

Taking it in turns, embark on a ceremony of body worship. Revere your lover's entire body as a physical manifestation of the god and goddess so that your every touch, caress, and kiss is filled with love. The man should worship his Shakti's body and scatter fragrant petals onto her yoni, revering it as the sacred gateway to sexual ecstasy. Then the woman can perform a similar ritual, touching her lover's body with deep veneration and spiritual devotion, scattering scented petals over his lingam.

"Shakti is the *essence of bliss;* she is the *love-power."*

DEVI PURANA

ACT 11: STILL COMMUNION

Whenever your mind takes you away from the moment, come back to your lover. Eye contact and synchronized breathing will take you deeper into your Tantric sexual experience. The scissor position shown here is perfect whenever you want to be joined in still, loving union.

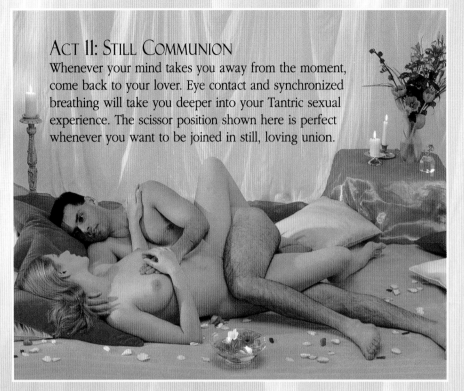

ACT 12: SACRED UNION

Begin to make love, letting every cell of your body flood with the joy of your kisses, embraces, and caresses. Enter the dimension of timelessness, hastening nowhere but surrendering yourselves into every exquisite sensation and impulse of the moment Synchronize breath and movement, merging together. In the Tantric sitting posture, known as Yab Yum (Mother-Father) in Buddhist Tantra, dissolve into ecstatic cosmic union. Become the Cosmic Lovers, Shiva and Shakti. Be as one.

> "After *merging* with each other, they ultimately dissolve in the *individual soul*" SHIVA PURANA

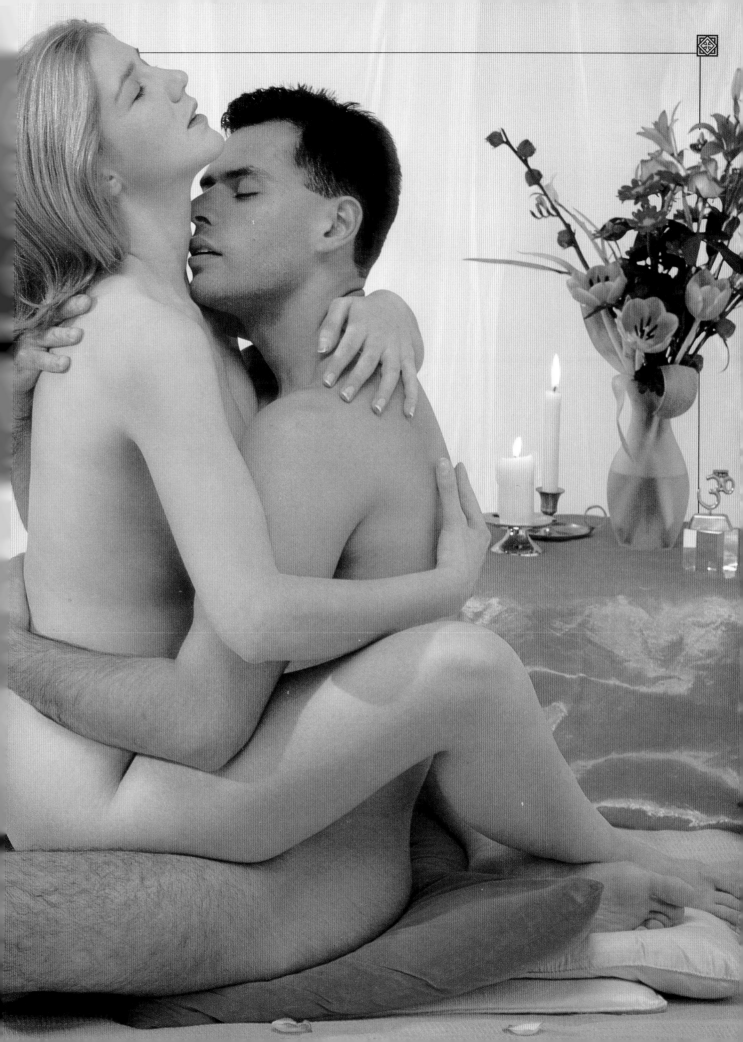

GLOSSARY

AJNA CHAKRA
The sixth chakra, located at a point between the eyebrows. Often referred to as the Third Eye, it is represented by a two-petaled lotus flower.

ANAHATA CHAKRA
The fourth chakra, which is located at the heart center. Its principle is air. It is represented by a twelve-petaled lotus flower.

ASANAS
Yogic postures that are employed to exercise the physical body, broaden mental faculties, and enhance spiritual capabilities.

ASTRAL BODY
The subtle or etheric body, containing prana, mind, intellect, and emotions.

BANDHAS
Yogic postures that constrict or lock particular physical organs and psychic energies. Employed by Tantrikas to aid the retention of semen.

CHAKRAS
The seven energy centers within the subtle body, each of which is visually represented by a form of lotus flower. The chakras correspond to nerve plexuses along the spine.

CHANDAMAHAROSANA
The Great Moon Elixir. The name of an important Tantra that is concerned with the control of lunar energy.

CHIN MUDRA
The yogic hand position made by joining the thumb and index finger.

DEVADASIS
Temple dancers, of whom several categories exist. Devadasis were the initiatresses of Tantra.

GUNAS
The three qualities of Nature: sattva, rajas, and tamas. According to yogic philosophy, everything is made up of the gunas in different proportions.

HATHA YOGA
The system of yoga that deals primarily with the physical body, using asanas as a means of harmonizing the breath and balancing solar and lunar energies.

IDA
One of three main nadis in the astral body. The subtle channel to the left of the Sushumna. From the left nostril it ascends to the crown of the head, then descends to the base of the spine.

KALI
The Hindu goddess of Transcendence, and the awesome aspect of Shakti. Transcendental sexual energy.

KUNDALINI
The latent psychosexual energy that, when awakened, rises up through the Sushumna. When correctly directed, Kundalini (or Kundalini Shakti) energy produces enlightenment.

LINGAM
The male sexual organ. Symbol of the Tantric god, Shiva. A phallic symbol.

MANDALA
A mystic circle that provides psychic protection during Tantric rituals.

MANIPURA CHAKRA
The third chakra, which is located in the region of the solar plexus. Its principle is fire. It is represented by a ten-petaled lotus flower.

MANTRA
A mystical syllable, word, or phrase, which is employed to focus the mind during meditation. Mantras can be repeated mentally or out loud.

MUDRA
A potent aid to Tantric meditation, th mystic hand gesture helps to produce psychic energy and channels prana in a specific direction.

MULADHARA CHAKRA
The lowest chakra, which is located at the base of the spine, between the anus and the sexual organs. Its principle is earth. It is represented visually by a four-petaled lotus.

NADIS
Channels that distribute psychic energ throughout the subtle body. The thre most important nadis are the Sushumn Ida, and Pingala.

NYASA
The touching of certain parts of the body to confer psychic protection during Tantric rituals. The process is usually accompanied by a mantra.

OM
The sacred syllable that symbolizes God, the Absolute Being. Sometimes written as Aum, Om is the universal mantra, containing the seed of all other mantras.

PADMASANA

[Th]e lotus posture. One of the most [im]portant asanas, it is a seated posture [wh]ere both legs are crossed and the [spi]ne is held erect. It is frequently [ad]opted as an aid to meditation.

PINGALA

[O]ne of three main nadis in the astral [bo]dy. The subtle channel to the right [of] the Sushumna. From the right nostril [it] ascends to the crown of the head, [th]en descends to the base of the spine.

PRANA

[T]he vital energy, or life force, flowing [th]rough the nadis of the subtle body.

PRANAYAMA

[B]reathing exercises designed to purify [a]nd strengthen the mind and body. [A]depts of pranayama can control the [fl]ow of prana in the body. The science [o]f prana is a potent aid to Liberation.

RADHA

[T]he presiding goddess of life energies, [r]epresenting success and achievement. [P]ersonified as the consort of Krishna.

RAJAS

[O]ne of the three gunas, rajas is the [q]uality of activity, mobility, and passion. [T]he arousing sentiment related to the [w]ill. Yogis traditionally avoid rajasic [c]onditions; Tantra transcends them.

SAHASRARA CHAKRA

The seventh chakra, symbolized by the thousand-petaled lotus flower. The highest chakra, it is here that the self unites with the cosmic whole.

SANSKRIT

Sanskrit is probably the most ancient human language. Tantra uses many Sanskrit terms because they cannot be translated precisely.

SATTVA

One of the three gunas, sattva is the quality of lightness and purity. The creative aspect of Nature, which leads to union with the Divine.

SHAKTI

The female creative energy and the kinetic force of Tantra. The primordial cosmic power personified by the great goddess, or Kundalini. The Mother of the Universe.

SHIVA

The divine inspiration of Tantra. Most of the secrets of Tantra are divulged in the form of a dialog between Shiva and his consort Parvati.

SHRI YANTRA

A mystic geometric diagram made up of five upward-pointing triangles and four downward-pointing triangles that symbolizes the cosmic union of the Tantric deities, Shiva and Shakti.

SHURYA

The Hindu Sun god, depicted as a golden figure riding a chariot drawn by seven horses. Tantrikas endeavor to awaken the energies of the inner sun, located in the navel region.

SUBTLE BODY

A yogic term that is used to describe the normally invisible psychic energy body that exists within and around the physical body. It is more commonly known as the astral body in the West.

SUSHUMNA

The principal energy channel in the subtle body, the most important of all the 72,000 nadis. It corresponds to the spinal chord in the physical body. The Sushumna connects this reality with a higher one. Pranic energy enters the Sushumna only during meditation.

SWADHISHTANA CHAKRA

The second energy junction along the Sushumna, it is located in the genital region. Represented by a six-petaled lotus, its principle is water.

TAMAS

One of the three gunas. The quality of lethargy, inertia, and ignorance. The destructive constituent of Nature.

TRANSCENDENTAL

The quality of going beyond the limitations of the mind. All meditation is transcendental by nature.

TRATAK

A purification gazing technique employed by Tantrikas to strengthen the eyes and stimulate latent powers of clairvoyance.

UPANISHADS

The great Sanskrit scriptures of ancient Hindu philosophy and religion.

VISHUDDHA CHAKRA

The fifth energy center in the subtle body. Located at the base of the throat, its principle is ether. It is represented by a sixteen-petaled lotus flower.

YANTRA

A mystic diagram used as a point of focus during meditation practices. Tantric sexual positions are described as yantras because they focus and channel energies.

YOGA

The communion of the individual self with the greater Self or godhead through a variety of means such as steadying postures and control of the vital breath.

YONI

The female sexual organ. Any symbol of this original source.

INDEX

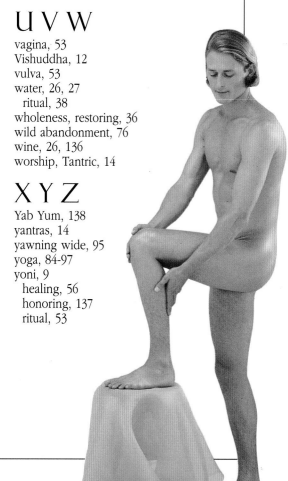

FURTHER READING

THE ART OF SEXUAL ECSTASY
Amand, Margo
The Aquarian Press, London, 1992

SEXUAL SECRETS
Douglas, Nik Slinger, Penny
Destiny Books, Rochester, 1979

THE TANTRIC WAY
Mookerjee, Ajit
Thames and Hudson, London, 1977

TANTRA (THE INDIAN CULT OF ECSTASY)
Rawson, Philip
Thames and Hudson, London, 1973

ACKNOWLEDGMENTS

AUTHOR'S ACKNOWLEDGMENTS
I would like to thank those who have taught and guided me to experience the ecstasy within. Thanks to Kevin Silous for his advice on Hatha Yoga. Special thanks to the models: George, Charlotte, Tariq, Susan, Michael, and Lucy.

DORLING KINDERSLEY WOULD LIKE TO
thank Fiona Wild for her invaluable editorial assistance and proofreading, Hilary Bird for compiling the index, all the models, and Barbara Launchbury for arranging their hair and make-up. Thank you also to Tamsin Pender for kind permission to photograph her phallic stone, and Pauline Clarke for illustrations on pages 12 and 13.

PICTURE CREDITS
All studio photography is by Mark Harwood. Dorling Kindersley would like to thank the following for their kind permission to reproduce photographs: Bridgeman Art Library/Fitzwilliam Museum, University of Cambridge p20; V&A Museum, London p32; ET Archive/V&A Museum, London p10; Werner Forman Archive Ltd./Philip Goldman Collection p6; Private Collection, N.Y. p98; Images Colour Library/Charles Walker Collection pp8, 16, 52, 84, 122; Pictor pp28-29; Thames and Hudson ©Photo John Webb, from *Tantra* by Philip Rawson pp13, 112.

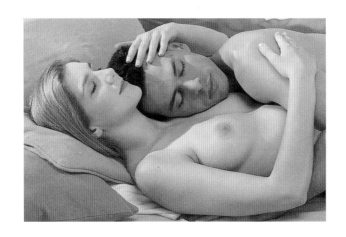